Eat
Yourself
Thin

Eat *Yourself* Thin

CHARLOTTE CARROLL

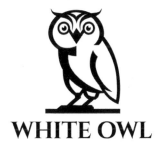

WHITE OWL

First published in Great Britain in 2017 by
WHITE OWL
an imprint of
Pen and Sword Books Ltd
47 Church Street
Barnsley
South Yorkshire S70 2AS

ISBN 978 1 47387 879 2

Printed and bound in Malta by
Gutenberg Press Ltd.

Pen & Sword Books Ltd incorporates the imprints of Pen & Sword
Archaeology, Atlas, Aviation, Battleground, Discovery, Family History,
History, Maritime, Military, Naval, Politics, Railways, Select, Social
History, Transport, True Crime, and Claymore Press, Frontline Books,
Leo Cooper, Praetorian Press, Remember When, Seaforth Publishing and
Wharncliffe.

For a complete list of Pen and Sword titles please contact
Pen and Sword Books Limited
47 Church Street, Barnsley, South Yorkshire, S70 2AS, England
E-mail: enquiries@pen-and-sword.co.uk
Website: www.pen-and-sword.co.uk

ACKNOWLEDGEMENTS

Firstly, I would like to thank you, the reader, for taking the first step towards changing your mind-set by purchasing this book.

Secondly, I would like to thank Heather Williams for giving me the opportunity to write this book and for all her help and support.

Finally, I would like to thank my partner, family and friends (especially the ones in the health and medical industry) for the support, advice and help given while researching and writing this book. You have all contributed to this with your confidence in me, and given me the push I needed to achieve another goal.

Thank you all!

CONTENTS

CHAPTER 1 - Confused about weight-loss?   11

Losing weight can seem a daunting process, but half the battle is preparation. This chapter shows how to prepare a programme that fits your lifestyle, including:

- ensuring you are ready for change
- setting short-term and long-term goals
- making a vision board
- assessing your eating habits
- keeping track of your progress with a food diary and an exercise log – both powerful tools on your weight-loss journey.

CHAPTER 2 - Understanding weight-loss   25

This is where we learn about calories, how they work and how to identify your optimum daily intake. I will also show you how to work out your BMI (body mass index) and BMR (basal metabolic rate) and how to use them to create an easy-to-follow plan.

CHAPTER 3 - Individual needs and components to a healthy diet   39

In this chapter we will look at the nutritional needs of adults, including vitamin and mineral intake, 5-a-day and, of course, the latest trends in dietary thinking.

CHAPTER 4 - Over-eating and how to overcome it?   57

In this chapter we will explore body image, methods of weight management and the ways positive thoughts can overcome negative thinking. We will also touch on weight-loss myths, which can overcomplicate some aspects of dieting.

CHAPTER 5 - Weight-loss vs life style change   75

This section will be useful for anyone who struggles with long-term diets. In it, I will explore different diet methods including: juicing, shake diets, supplements and physical exercise. I will list the positive aspects for each diet and explain how they can work for different people. This chapter will also look at diets from around the world and contains some great ideas and inspiration.

INTRODUCTION

Imagine this: a friend is watching you weigh yourself on the bathroom scales. She can see you pulling faces and says, 'try again without your socks on,' to which you don't know whether to laugh or cry. Does that sound familiar? Do you feel as if you've tried every diet there is? Don't worry, we've all been there. So many of my clients told me scales were their enemy, that I started to think up other methods I could use to change the way they felt about their weight, body image and, of course, food. Then it came to me: if many people struggle with diets that ask us to change our lifestyles and the food we consume, how about changing our attitudes instead. I don't mean we should change who we are as individuals, just that we could develop a positive attitude that works for each of us! And that's what I hope to achieve for YOU: I want to change your mind set to a positive one, because once you think positively then positive things will happen around you. By the end of this book you will have changed your outlook on food and appreciate what good nutrition does for the human body. So you are not just going on a diet to lose weight – YOU are going on a lifestyle journey!

Each year a new diet comes out and, along with it, another book. So I did wonder whether I should be adding to an already over-crowded market, then I realised that these diets come and go; what does not change is the medical advice to consume less fat and sugar and to do more exercise. If these diets worked, we would all be happy and healthy and slim BUT we are not. These books are not answering our questions or giving us the advice we need to achieve our goals. I know that good nutrition is the key to change, but we need educating if we hope to see the positive changes I want to implement.

What will you gain from following this book? Not only will you lose weight, you will get lots more energy, strong immunity from endless sniffling colds and coughs, better concentration, glowing skin and hair and improved circulation. You will gain a positive mental attitude and be ready to smash some personal goals! Instead of looking at what you need to give up, think about what you will gain.

Each chapter breaks down the principles you may have previously found hard to understand. Each chapter contains HUMOUR and the MOTIVATION to help you on your journey. What is even better is that you can do all of it from the comfort of your own home: in the bath, cooking the dinner – you may even be finishing the ironing with this book in one hand.

It may contain the dreaded weigh-in and it may contain ways of achieving your goal you've not thought of before but, with my help and support, it WILL help you develop into the person you want become – which is a few pounds lighter!

Let us start our journey together and take a look at what we have to explore in the world of weight-loss.

CHAPTER 1
CONFUSED ABOUT WEIGHT-LOSS?

WHY DO WE EAT?

This may seem like a simple question and you're probably thinking: because we are hungry! But it is actually a serious one, which needs to be explored in more detail. Sometimes we eat without even realising it's happening! We can eat through boredom, habit or to comfort ourselves emotionally. Sometimes, for example at special occasions, we eat out of politeness. We put weight on because we are eating the wrong foods. Maybe you have a medical condition, which causes weight gain, or are taking medication which gives the same result, or maybe you have issues with food and you can't help yourself. Do any of these sound familiar? We will go through some of them later in the book and look at how we can break our eating habits – we will even discuss the struggle of eating out. Initially, though, we need to explore what a diet is and what we mean by healthy diets.

WHAT IS A DIET?

A diet is simply the food we eat. It can be healthy or unhealthy, carnivorous or vegetarian, restricted by regional availability or broad enough to include food from all over the world. Some people follow a specific type of diet due to a medical condition or for religious reasons – if this is you, please talk to your doctor before starting your weight-loss journey as he or she will help you balance your nutritional requirements.

For most people, however, diet means a weight-loss programme. This isn't wrong, but I prefer to call this kind of diet, a weight-loss journey. I find that when people choose to lose weight, it is not for a short period of time – unless they are crash dieters.

Crash dieters are those who lose weight quickly for a holiday or special occasion and then moan, when it piles back on, that the diet hasn't worked. It won't, as they are not trying to maintain the results.

Those who choose to turn their journey into a lifestyle change want see long-term benefits to their bodyshape and health. They understand that weight-loss is not the two-week fix some diets out there claim, sustained weight-loss is changing how you think about food, the way you cook it and what you want to accomplish and maintain.

However we define diet, it is about making our own choices, about what we put in our mouths and, in the case of weight-loss, the specific eating plan we follow to achieve this.

Having a good diet means consuming the right balance of nutrients and not overeating. I am here to help you figure out the best weight-loss journey to meet your needs.

WHY DIETS DON'T WORK?

Diets don't work for a variety of reasons. Sometimes its because they ignore the rules of proper nutrition, leaving you hungry or nutritionally imbalanced, which leads to cheating. Sometimes they ask you to eliminate so many food groups or meals, they are simply unsustainable. Or maybe your willpower isn't there when temptation is. Could these reasons be why a diet didn't work for you? Write down what has caused you to fail on previous weight-loss journeys and then what you want to achieve on this one. Comparing the two should give you an understanding and awareness of what you need to do differently and how you need to do it. This will be part of your planning and preparation. Keep the lists and take a look when you have finished this book to see how your attitudes have changed. Think of this book as a journey to good nutrition. I want you to learn, I want you to understand and most of all I want you to achieve.

CONFUSED ABOUT WEIGHT-LOSS?

Do you get confused about conflicting nutritional advice?

It seems that one day we are told specific foods are bad for us, then the next we are told they are good. If you asked people to tell you about 'good' and 'bad' foods, you would probably get a variety of responses. Some might say that bread is bad, or that you need a low-carb diet because carbs are bad. Others would say you should stay away from fats, even though some dieticians argue that some fats are good for you. There is evidence that eating dairy foods aids weight-loss, while the debate continues in the media and online about whether foods such as chocolate and red wine are part of a healthy diet. If we listened to every opinion, we wouldn't eat anything. So who should we trust? I'd advise that, in addition to this book, you find a reliable source and stick with it. You won't go wrong with the dietary advice from the government – try the Food and Diet section at www.nhs.uk. I would trust sensible guidelines, backed by proper research over an article on a blog any day.

Hands up if you have tried diet crazes, which promise 'guaranteed results' and the body and lifestyle of a supermodel in a week. You know, the ones you give up because they don't work? I have been there, my mum has, my friends have – even my grandmother has. So if this applies to you, then you are not alone. Any diet will work if it helps you take in fewer calories, but if it doesn't offer balanced nutrition, or is too extreme, then it will be unsustainable in the longrun. I believe, clean eating is the best way to lose weight and maintain those results.

Most of us know what a healthy diet looks like – even if we don't we can easily find out from government guidelines and medical advice – why don't we just follow one? Possibly because we so busy caring for our families, pursuing our careers, helping out our friends and sharing time with others. We are all busy bees in today's society, so it is easy to lose sight of what makes a healthy lifestyle. Whatever the reason behind your struggle to lose weight, I have written this book to help YOU achieve results through basic guidance. What may seem complicated at the start will make sense by the end and hopefully change how you think about and behave with food.

So now you know what this book is about, let us get started. You have identified that you would like to lose weight or make a healthy change to your lifestyle, so you have made your first step. Now I will go through some simple steps on how to plan so your hard work will pay off.

First of all, I will discuss your BMI and BMR, also known as your body mass index and basal metabolic rate, as these alone can give people the motivation they need to start their journey. To work out your BMI I like to follow an online tool, which calculates whether you are underweight, healthy, overweight or obese, and then determines the weight range for your build. Your BMI is calculated on your gender, age, height and your weight.

'Your BMI allows for natural variations in body shape, giving a healthy weight range for a particular height. The calculation divides the adult's weight in kilograms by their height in metres and squared.' (NHS, 2013)

You can find an online tool to work out your BMI by typing 'what is my body mass index?' into any search engine and clicking on a reliable source. If you do not have access to the internet, speak to your GP as they will be able to help you work this out. Your BMI will give you a starting point on your weight-loss journey and help you determine whether you need to gain or lose weight and by how much. Write it down as this will help you monitor your achievements on the way.

A BMI of less than 18 is classed as underweight, between 18 and 25 is defined as healthy, over 25 is overweight and over 30 is obese. Do not be nervous if you see the words 'overweight' or 'obese' when working out your BMI. This is just a recommendation and it will help prepare you for your tasks and goals ahead.

Obesity is defined in many ways but, unless the cause is medical, it is nothing that you cannot overcome and change. You may feel mortified when you hear you are classed as obese, but it is estimated that one in four adults in the UK are classed as obese, usually because they eat too much and don't do enough exercise. This is nothing that cannot solved with the right attitude. Banish negative thoughts: it is time to get positive and believe that you can do this! Labelling someone as obese can feel humiliating, but I would use this 'label' to set some targets and smash some personal goals.

Try some affirmations – these are positive statements, which help us focus on our good points instead of being dragged down by negative thinking. Examples include:

> **I have a beautiful smile.**
> **I look great in red.**
> **I am very stylish.**

Write down some positive messages and say them to yourself every day while you are cleaning your teeth, driving your car, or waiting for the bus etc.

Do not look at this programme as a diet, think of it as permanent lifestyle change which will benefit your whole life, your weight, your health, your nutrition, your mind, your mood and your behaviours and attitudes towards food and drink.

ARE YOU ARE READY?

Do you know why you would like to lose weight? Maybe you want to look or feel better, maybe it's for health reasons or just to feel physically enhanced. Write down your reasons and any health benefits of weight-loss, why you want to lose weight and how you plan to do this.

You may be feeling mixed emotions. Are you nervous, anxious, terrified, daunted or maybe excited, motivated and positive? However you feel, planning your healthy lifestyle change is the key to a productive journey. Planning is not only about organising your foods, drink and exercise, it is also about recognising and evaluating old habits, short- and long-term goals, keeping track of your progress and preparing mentally. Your weight-loss journey will be based on willpower and eliminating old habits from your routine.

Willpower is the ability to control your own thoughts and impulses.

You may have tried weight-loss in the past and failed, however this does not mean that you will fail every time. Maybe you didn't assess your lifestyle and identify clearly what really needs to change, or maybe you set yourself unrealistic targets and goals. The main tool when setting a target for change is willpower – whether it's weight-loss or giving up smoking.

So the first step is ensuring you are mentally prepared by giving yourself a mental makeover!

It's not a diet
ITS CALLED EATING HEALTHY

Step 1

Let us look at what type of weight-loss personality you are? Dr Thomas R. Przybeck of Washington University School of Medicine, St Louis, believes that personality plays a huge role in our attitude towards food and there are five types:

Impulsive – if you are unable to control your thoughts and cravings and tend to eat the wrong foods at the wrong time with no thoughts or consideration of the consequences, then this is you. You need to remove yourself from temptation.

Oblivious – are you unaware of, or do not pay attention to, what you eat? For example, do you snack while watching TV?

Uptight – emotional eaters eat in response to feelings such as anxiety, nervousness or depression. Binge eating comes in this category, as bingeing is a response to a negative emotion and will often make you feel better.

Tenacious – some people have no trouble at all losing weight once they set their minds to it. If this is you then you will have an easier time.

Sociable – you are good at monitoring your food intake especially in social surroundings, for example while out with family and friends, or taking a lunch break at work.

Can you relate to any of these personalities? Which one? Write down some of the habits around food that put you in this category. Then write down some things you could do to change them.

Step 2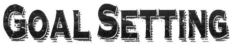

Goal setting! You need to set short- and long-term goals. They need to be realistic and achievable. If you don't set sensible goals, the more likely you will be to give up on your journey. Think of it as an adventure and when you hit your goals, the more determined you will be to achieve new ones. When setting goals, think of what will keep you motivated. Pin them up on the fridge or put post-it notes on your wall where you can see them. When I set goals for myself I like to think of the ways I can achieve them. I have them on the wall in my bedroom. Sometimes I put funny pictures on my fridge to make me laugh and keep me motivated. Think of little non-food based rewards to give yourself when you achieve one.

Short-term goals

A short-term goal is something you want to accomplish in the near future, maybe within a week, month or three months. Short-term goals are the small steps of planning that lead to long-term success. They are much easier to visualise, so writing down the actions you need to take to achieve them will bring you that step closer to your long-term aim.

Examples of short-term goals: I want to increase my exercise levels within the first week of my journey. I will achieve this by walking to work each day rather than driving.

I want to increase my activity levels within the first two weeks. I will start by jogging once within my first week for fifteen minutes. In my second week I will increase this by another fifteen minutes.

In order for me to be realistic I will decrease the amount of snacks I consume through the day. On my first day I'll swap biscuits for fruit.

I want to achieve a healthier lifestyle; to attain this I will swap less healthy foods for healthier ones. I will grill my food instead of frying it. I want to lose 6lb (2.5kg) in a month through healthy eating and gentle exercise.

Not only will you feel a momentum build by writing down these goals, they will keep you focused. They are a quick and effective way to build up your confidence and achieve meaningful objectives. They will help you remain positive.

Long-term goals

Long-term goals are what you would like to accomplish the distant future. This could be in six months, a year or longer. Long-term goals must be attainable and you reach them by accomplishing your short-term healthy eating and exercise goals. Long-term goals help you keep going if you miss one of your short-term goals.

Examples of long-term goals: Within six months of my weight-loss journey I would like to have lost two stone (13kg).

After attending the gym and exercising regularly, I would like to run a marathon next year. I have enjoyed the gym so much I am going to sign up for three more classes within the next six months.

Now I have achieved my short-term goals of healthy eating and made a permanent lifestyle change, I will reassess my healthy eating every three months to maintain it.

Long-term goals may take more dedication and perseverance, however they become more realistic and achievable when you are enthusiastic and committed.

____ WHAT TO THINK ABOUT WHEN SETTING GOALS ____

The SMART goal tool will help you realise your goals whether short or long-term. SMART stands for Specific, Measured, Attainable, Realistic and Time-bound – think about these when you are setting your goals.

Specific

The more specific you can be the better as the goal will be much easier to hit. Ask:

Who? – who will help you reach it? Who will support you? Who can give you guidance?

This could be your GP, nutritionist, partner, family, friends or maybe a support group. Or it could also just be you. You may choose to look at this as not only a goal but also a project: Project Me you could call it. You could research all your own information – always using reliable sources.

What? – what are you going to do to reach your ideal weight? What will you change? What are your bad habits?

These are changes that will help you: doing more exercise, making diet plans, clearing fatty and sugary foods out of the fridge and cupboards. Write down your bad habits then think about what you can do to change them. Focus on any barriers and what you could do to overcome them.

Where – where will you achieve your weight-loss? Where will you complete your goals? Where will you shop?

These are some of the places that will help you achieve weight-loss: gym, home, supermarkets, local shops, farmers' markets. What will the changes cost you? Think about ways to do your shopping that will avoid temptation and keep costs down.

When – When will you set your target dates? When are you going to start?

Setting target dates is important but so is setting targets that are realistic.

So don't put them too close together. Steer clear of aiming too high, which could cause you to fall at the first hurdle. Just stay consistent.

Why – Why are you choosing to do this? Why are you setting targets?

Your reasons for setting goals can be a real eye - opener and also a massive motivator. Weight-loss is usually the first goal, but how about adding other features such as better health, positive attitude, clearer skin? The choices are endless.

How – How will you achieve goals? How will you feel when you have achieved them?

Think about the planning and preparation – if you are clear about what you want to achieve your journey will be easier. Give yourself a reward each time you reach a goal and then think of ways you can move it on. For example, if you completed two workouts one week, try three the following week; or if you cooked three healthy meals one week try four in the next. The feelings of success, achievement and happiness you'll experience will be your biggest inspiration and give you the drive to aim higher.

Measurable

You will need to measure your progress in order to obtain your goal. This can be done either by weighing yourself or measuring inches (or centimetres) lost around your waist, thighs, hips. This does not mean weigh yourself every day! Aim for once a week. Measurements should be documented within your goals.

Attainable

Your goals must be attainable but also challenging: remember recommended weight-loss is no more than 2lb (1kg) a week. If your targets are not realistic, then you will lose heart and be more likely to quit. If you think this applies to you, take a moment to reset them.

Relevant

You need goals that are relevant to you. If they are not relevant, then you will not be motivated to achieve them. For example, if you don't like running or jogging then do not set a goal that involves running. If you can't swim don't make a goal to swim for half an hour each week. The more relevant the goal is to you as a person, the easier it will be and greater the effort you will make to achieve it. For example, if you enjoy cycling then maybe you could do more and possibly join a cycling group.

TIME

Having deadlines makes it easier to focus on goals, but make sure they, are planned around your lifestyle and again make sure they are realistic. This about YOU controlling your programme, not the programme controlling you.

You need ensure you are planning correctly. This includes:

Being Honest – Can you cook? Will you cook? Do you have time to prepare healthy meals each night? Do you like exercising? If not, and you set exercise as a goal, you might find excuses not to do it. Are there specific foods you do not enjoy? If so, plan meals that don't include them. Be honest about how you will overcome any obstacles? Buy a calendar, notebook or download an app to your smart phone and use it to set dates for your goals.

Planning your cheat meals in advance is a big help. It is inevitable that you will have meals out or social events to attend. Put all these on your calendar so you can plan your weight-loss meals around them and keep cravings under control, that way you won't feel like you have failed. Everyone is entitled to a cheat day, so don't panic if you treat yourself. It's not the end of the world!

After making a list of your goals, set yourself rewards. For example, when you reach your first milestone treat yourself to a beauty treatment. Reward yourself each time you reach a target, but not with clothes. Clothes can have a negative impact if you still do not fit into them. Instead, buy a new pair of running shoes or a bicycle when you reach a big target. This instantly gives you more motivation and determination to succeed.

Step 3

Body vision boards

I find these help so many people focus. Studies have shown that pictures have the ability to make us feel more positive. Since losing weight is the point of your whole focus, visualising yourself in better shape creates a platform for the way you want to look. Imagination is the greatest tool for weight-loss so you need a clear vision of what you would like to look like: aim for an ideal weight based on your height, frame and age and not on unhealthy images you see in the media.

Write down how you look now, then on another page write down what you want to look like. Be specific.

Then create the vision by cutting photographs from magazines of people with the weight, hairstyle or clothes you would like. Copy and stick these on to a big poster and place this on your wall to look at each day. If you're up on technology, you can use an application on your smart phone to do this. Make it the screensaver on your phone or computer so you see it every day. Doing this will etch your ideal into your subconscious mind and this will help you create your ideal body image. Positive body image will be discussed with in Chapter 4 but examples could include: I'm a size 8 with a firm butt and toned arms. I am full of energy and feel healthier than ever before. I have incredible fitness and stamina! I am a size 12 with toned abs. The energy I am feeling right now and my healthy diet makes me feel amazing.

Visualise your fridge! Yes, really, your fridge! Look at the contents, then draw a picture of how it will look filled with healthy food. Think colourful fruits and salads with fresh meats and fish and bottles of water instead of alcohol.

You can refer back to this at the end of your journey and see if your fridge matches the drawing.

Step 4

Learning to control your habits is vital. Breaking old behaviours to make way for new ones can be difficult, but this is essential to good planning. A habit is there for a reason and it somehow has a benefit to your life whether good or bad. Learning how to control and replace bad habits is key to overcoming them. So, if the first thing you do when you wake up is cook a bacon sandwich then try changing this to having a shower or turning on the TV – this is called using a trigger. A trigger is what you do before you form a habit so a trigger will help you form a new pattern. Alternatively, you could use this time to complete exercises or go for a walk.

Evening habits can be the hardest to break. Clear out any fatty snacks you might be tempted to munch on while watching TV and replace them with healthy ones – I'll give ideas later. You always need to replace one habit with another as you need to satisfy the need it fulfils. So if you wind down each night with a glass of wine, chocolates or cheese and crackers, why not swap this for going to the gym, doing a DVD workout or even reading books which may help and guide you.

There is scientific proof that bad habits can be broken and it is not difficult if you are willing to stick with the method for a month. Here's a summary:

1. Determine the bad habit you want to break by identifying the problem.
2. Write it down.
3. Identify your triggers and the replacement strategies you could use to overcome them.
4. Make a series of stickers with positive reinforcements on them and tape or place them so you can see them all day long, even at your desk.

Make the stickers using POSITIVE language, not negative. For instance: 'Today, I am healthy and I stay away from fatty foods.'

5. Repeat the phrase several times a day. Use music or other positive reinforcements to enhance the technique.

6. **Focus on replacement habits** – instead of reaching for a bar of chocolate, have fruit nearby to snack on.

7. Keep this routine for thirty straight days, no cheating. This should help break the habit – repeat it for other habits you want to change.

Write down the new habits as this will help you ease yourself into the new routine. Draw on visualisation to help you. Don't forget to give yourself time to change and if you slip up, just start again. Cravings will come and go, so have tactics in place to help you overpower them.

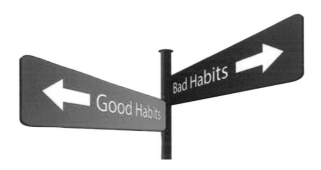

Step 5

Now it is time to think about menu planning and food preparation. There are a number of different ways that you can cook and prepare your foods. Some of these methods will be healthier than others.

The areas to consider are food selection, cooking methods, the utensils and storage boxes you will use to help you stick to the right portion sizes. Also, consider cooking times. If you have a busy lifestyle, then you might think healthy eating is time consuming. Many people have said this to me and my answer is planning. If you cook every day, why not prepare the food before work (this is where slow cookers are amazing inventions). Set aside time at the weekend or mid-week to prepare all your meals for the week and freeze them. Then all you need to do is defrost the meal when you need it and pop it in the oven. Lunches are easy to prepare the night before if you are having salad or maybe try making soup and refrigerating the leftovers for lunch the next day. Don't skip breakfast. People often mistakenly think this will help them shed pounds more quickly when, in fact, breakfast really is the most important meal of the day. Healthy and nutritious breakfasts can be simple and quick. If you don't like certain foods, then you need to overcome this by thinking of alternatives. For example, if you are a vegetarian you need to find ways of getting enough protein in your healthy and balanced diet. I will discuss food options and alternatives later in the chapter but you need to be aware of this at the planning stage.

Cooking utensils may not seem obvious until you think about how you cook your food? I would steer away from frying as steaming, grilling or baking are better. They preserve more of the food nutrients and don't involve extra fat. If you wish to fry, use alternative, healthier, oils such as coconut. Invest in a blender or hand blender to make delicious homemade smoothies or soups. A set of scales or measuring cups will ensure you keep control of your portion sizes. Storage boxes are also handy, especially if you are keen to prepare food in advance. As simple as it sounds, being so organised will help you massively and give you a real sense of satisfaction.

Simple changes can make all the difference!

Step 6

Keeping track of progress is essential!

This DOES NOT MEAN WEIGH YOUR SELF DAILY! Weighing yourself daily will only have a negative impact. Healthy eating and losing weight is a lifestyle change and takes time.

You could purchase scales and, yes, monitor your weight once a week or maybe every two weeks, but the most effective way of monitoring weight-loss is by measuring the size of your body. This includes neck, chest, upper arms, waist, thighs, calves and ankles. Remain positive throughout this. You may not lose pounds straight away but once you feel your clothes loosening, you'll get the focus and determination to achieve. You could even make a dartboard and put your target weight on it.

When you have a balanced and healthy diet you feel good, have plenty of energy and avoid a number of health risks. There is no one food plan that suits everybody as everyone is different. We all have slightly different nutritional requirements, depending on a number of different factors which will be discussed further on. However you will all lose weight if you follow the eating and exercise regime that suits you best.

Keeping a food log is important to your planning as it gives you an idea of what you are eating and drinking and so what you need to change. The same goes for exercise – if you are working out then this needs to be documented so you can look at what you may need to alter. I have included an example of an exercise and food diary later on to help you. It is imperative that you keep track of this whether you are writing it on your smart phone, paper or calendar. If it helps, purchase a little book or diary and fill it with motivational quotes and pictures. On the first page, write down ten things you like about yourself – keep looking them and reminding yourself. All this is part of visualisation. For example, you might not notice you are eating five biscuits a night in front of the TV, but when you record it you will realise that this is not healthy and that things need to change. If you are dreaming of chocolate to the point where your mouth is watering, then give yourself an alternative option such as a shake. Add some flavouring to take the cravings away. I also find dark chocolate made of more than 70 per cent cocoa is a good snack – it's not so high in sugar and its intensity means you can only eat a small amount at a time.

This chapter should have you ready to start your preparation. Just keep one thing in mind – when you feel like quitting, remember why you started.

The next chapter is based on calories and elements we need for a healthy lifestyle.

CHAPTER 2

CALORIES AND COMPONENTS TO A HEALTHY DIET

'If you are persistent you will get it, if you are consistent you will keep it'

I call this chapter the humdrum chapter as it's all about the confusing and tedious stuff that can put you off even starting a healthy eating plan. But it is simple once it's been explained in a straightforward way. Many people do not believe in calorie counting. I don't believe you should count daily, but you do need to be aware of what your calorie intake should be, and which foods contain the most calories, or you will continue to eat snacks which you think are fine when in fact they are helping you pile on more weight. It is not being a calorie bore, it is being realistic and sensible about the foods you are eating.

It's 2017, why does food still have calories

———— LET'S GET EXCITED ABOUT CALORIES! ————

'Calories are tiny creatures that live in your closet and sew your clothes a little bit tighter each night.' Right? I wish they were as then we may be able to get rid of them quicker.

However, it is not quite as easy as that. Let us start with the question: what do we need food for? We need food to give our bodies energy. It's that simple! A calorie is one unit of energy. The human body receives energy from food in the form of calories. Food contains calories and these come from carbohydrates, fats and proteins. They can be measured in ounces or grammes:

0.03oz (1g) of carbs = 4 calories
0.03oz (1g) of protein = 4 calories
0.03oz (1g) of fat = 9 calories

Don't be confused – this is the simplest way of writing it down. I can explain further how to calculate these measurements!

There is a debate about whether calculating calories is the best way to monitor food intake and some people choose to count colours. What do they mean by this? They believe that counting the colours of your food and drink is the best way to lose weight as each food colouring is beneficial to a person. This will be discussed further, later in the book.

So what do we use calories for? We use calories not just for energy such as walking and running, but also talking, breathing and even sleeping. So when you are asleep you are actually burning those dreaded things that cause weight gain. Great eh? However, I don't advise that you sleep throughout the day and night just to shift these calories, although it would be fantastic if we could. Here's an example, if you CONSUME 3,500 calories more than you USE you will gain 1lb (0.45g) in body fat but, if you USE 3,500 calories more than you CONSUME then you would lose 1lb (0.45g) of body fat.

So how many calories should a person consume? I believe that this calculation should be based on your body mass index (BMI) and basal metabolic tate (BMR) since every person is different in height, size and shape. These are two entirely different but essential measurements that are really useful in helping with weight-loss. Your BMI, as we have seen, is calculated on your height and weight and used to work out how much fat in your body. The classifications are underweight, normal weight, overweight and obese. It is only a very general measurement as it doesn't take into account muscle mass, gender or age. So don't worry if your BMI is high, the more you exercise you do and the more muscle mass you have, the more calories you will need to consume to maintain your weight. Older adults have a lower BMI than younger people and this is simply due to muscle mass decreasing with age.

Your BMR works out the number of calories your body needs just to function and represents between 40 and 70 per cent of your daily energy requirement, depending on age and lifestyle. The factors that determine this are genes, body composition and activity levels. The average calorie requirement for men is 2,550 and a woman 2,000 but this varies depending on your age, level of activity and how much weight you want to lose. This does not mean eating nothing at all, it means swapping your bad foods for healthy ones thereby reducing your calorie intake on bad fats and sugary foods.

You should know your BMI and BMR as they can help you to keep a better track of the calories you should be consuming.

If you really want to know how to measure your BMI, divide your weight in pounds by the square of your height in inches then multiply by 703.

The sum looks like this: weight ÷ (height x height) x 703

However, you'll be relieved to know there are online calculators to work it out for you. Don't forget to find a reputable one like the one on the NHS website.

To work out your BMR look for the Harris Benedict equation online and find a calculator from a trustworthy website to help you – good old NHS again. The equations are different for women and men. The table below shows how this is worked out:

Harris Benedict Formula

To determine your total daily calorie needs, multiply your BMR by the appropriate activity factor, as follows:

If you are sedentary (little or no exercise):
Calorie-Calculation = **BMR x 1.2**

If you are lightly active (light exercise/sports 1-3 days/week):
Calorie-Calculation = **BMR x 1.375**

If you are moderately active (moderate exercise/sports 3-5 days/week):
Calorie-Calculation = **BMR x 1.55**

If you are very active (hard exercise/sports 6-7 days a week):
Calorie-Calculation = **BMR x 1.725**

If you are extra active (very hard exercise/sports and physical job or 2x training):

Calorie-Calculation = **BMR x 1.9**

So you would complete the formula as shown below:

BMR X PAL = TOTAL ENERGY REQUIRMENT

So next, work out your physical activity levels. It doesn't matter if you're unable to complete certain types of exercise due, for example, to medical problems. This is fine and you should never feel less motivated because of this. Obviously the higher your level of activity, the more energy you need to burn. To work this out we go back to the Harris Benedict equation. A person's physical activity level (PAL) is determined by what he/she does in a twenty-four-hour period.

Barriers such as jobs, social life, children, disability and medical conditions can affect our ability to get fitter but most of us can make simple but effective changes to improve our physical activity levels. Just half an hour a day is three and a half hours a week. Once you have worked out your total energy requirement, write it down and let's start thinking about how we can apply it to our eating habits.

So are you ready now to burn some calories? Every time I think of burning calories, I think of a gym class, which will cause me days of pain from aching muscles, but in reality all you need is to work out your recommended calorie intake and how many you need to burn in order to keep a healthy weight! You might only need to make small changes such as swapping driving for walking to work or taking the kids to the park instead of to a fast food restaurant, which is where children usually prefer to go. Making these activities fun is half the battle!

Food labelling

Calories are shown on food labels, which is one reason reading nutritional labelling is so important. We live in a busy society in which processed foods and ready meals are the easier and more convenient choice, but they are also a huge barrier to healthy eating. And many people do not read the packaging since, to them, food shopping is a chore just like housework and ironing.

Imagine this, a mum takes her two children to the local supermarket, she is stressed out, the shop is busy, she wants to get back to watch her favourite soap opera then one of her children notices the toy aisle, both children are now in the toy aisle and fighting over a toy. Do you think this lady wants to shop now, never mind check the nutritional labelling on the packaging of food?

It has been a legal requirement since 1996 for the majority of food products sold in the UK and internationally, including processed and pre-prepared foods, to carry nutritional information labels. This is to prevent false advertising, promote food safety and ensure food quality. It is to help YOU, the buyer, to make informed decisions about the food you are consuming. If a product's packaging simply states the name and brief description of what the product is, for example, 'this apple pie is filled with real apples and tastes delicious,' then this is impossible to make a sensible judgement about its nutritional value. You might think, and not unreasonably, that it is all right to have as a treat, but without more information, how do you know? Certain products, such as beef, fish, fruit and vegetables, olive oil and poultry, must show their county or origin since they can be imported from outside the European Union (EU). However there is an exception: food that is sold loose, such as fruit and vegetables, is exempt from many of the regulations. The items that must, by law, be displayed on the label are:

Manufacturer's name and contact details
Name of the product
Description

Weight – though some foods, such as bread, are exempt from this

The ingredients if there are more than two

Cooking and heating instructions

Special storage conditions

Shelf life

Place of origin – since certain food and drinks are imported from outside the EU

Allergy information and warnings such as 'Not suitable for...'

In addition there will be information about the nutritional value of your food

– the amount of fat, protein, carbohydrates, salts, sugar and vitamins it contains. It is important to read this in order to keep your diet balanced and your sugar and salt intake to a minimum. At the moment, nutritional labelling is optional and only compulsory if a food manufacturer makes a nutritional claim about food such as 'low in fat' or 'low in sugar' or if vitamins and minerals have been added. Manufacturers have to follow the EU rules for nutritional labelling. From December 2016, all this information will need to be stipulated for all pre-packed products and must show:

The energy value of food in kilojoules and kilocalories

The amount of fat, protein and carbohydrates in grammes

Any additional information relating to a nutritional claim being made

Values should be given per 100g, per 100ml and per packet or portion

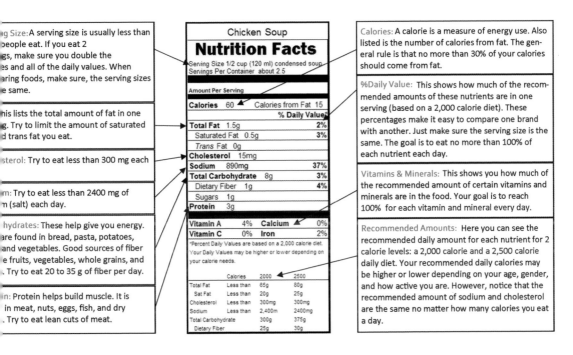

Products which make a statement or suggestion that a relationship exists between food and health, such as 'helps support immunity', or that the product can improve

a person's health in a specific way, such as 'helps reduce digestive discomfort', must follow further guidelines and the claim must be understandable to the average customer. The claims should be honest and truthful and not misleading and apply to food after it has been prepared according to the packet instructions. Medical claims that a product can prevent, treat or cure a disease are not allowed on food labelling, neither are any claims that your health could be affected by not consuming the product. Other claims not permitted on food labels are any references to the rate or amount of weight-loss as a direct result of consuming the product or endorsements from individual doctors or health professionals. Nor should the manufacturer ever question the safety and nutritional content of other foods when promoting or advertising their own. The claims must be easy, and well–defined, for the customer to understand.

Food labelling and food inspections date back to 1906 and the USA when the Food and Drugs and Federal Meat Inspection Act was introduced. Since then further legislation worldwide has resulted in the introduction of recommended daily intakes, guideline daily amounts. More recently reference intakes were introduced by our government to provide people with simple, reliable information on food and nutrition. Most labels have reference intakes on them, which show what proportion a particular serving is in relation your recommended daily intake. It is also informs us how much saturated fat and salt is considered healthy so we can make informed decisions about the products we are buying.

So how are reference intakes measured? Unless the label states otherwise, they are based on an average-sized woman doing a consistent amount of physical activity. This is to help those with lower energy requirements reduce the risk of overeating as well as providing clear and consistent information on labels. These guidelines are for an average person of healthy weight but are based on those set for women to avoid over consumption.

The NHS stated that an adult's reference intakes for a day are:

Energy: 8,400kJ/2,000kcal
Total fat: 70g
Saturates: 20g
Carbohydrate: 260g
Total sugars: 90g
Protein: 50g
Salt: 6g

If you are trying to lose weight, your daily energy requirement will be lower than if you want your weight to remain stable. This is where your BMR comes in as knowing this will help you work out how many calories you need to consume to help you lose weight the healthy way. Why is there a limit on fats, sugars and salt? These three things can cause obesity, which can then lead to health problems such as a stroke, heart disease, diabetes and tooth decay. Not good. Monitoring how much fat, sugar and salt you are consuming is a massive part of having a healthy diet, which is why the food labels can be so important in helping you achieve this.

Sugars

Sugars provide energy, however it is very easy to have too much sugar by eating lots of little treats such as chocolate and cakes. Finding the sugar guidelines is easy – just look for the carbohydrate figure on the food label. Added sugars should not make up more than 5 per cent of the energy that you get from drink and food daily. This approximately works out at around 30g a day for those aged eleven and over. We are always being told to cut back on sugar, but why is it so bad for us? Well, we know it rots teeth, adds weight and causes obesity, but it can also increase your chances of getting type 2 diabetes and heart disease. White sugar does not contain any nutrients either, while brown sugar contains low levels of minor minerals. Sweets and manufactured food products filled with sugar are readily available and also cheap, which is one reason people think healthy eating is expensive in comparison. But sugar does not just exist in cakes, drinks and chocolate, it is also added to cereals, tinned beans, spaghetti, sauces and other processed foods. According to the BBC, 'sugar consumption is at its highest level in history. Global consumption of added sugar has increased by a whopping 46 per cent per person per day in the last thirty years.' That is one big sugar rush. Recently there have been debates around fruit and how fruit is bad for us because of the sugar it contains. I don't see the relevance in comparing fruit to a chocolate bar as the fruit contains vital nutrients, a chocolate bar does not. Let me explain.

Fruit contains a natural sugar called fructose. So if sugar is bad for us, and it's in fruit, why are we advised to eat fruit? More importantly, why are diabetics encouraged to do it if it poses a risk? Unlike sucrose, or refined sugars, fructose does not cause sudden instabilities in your blood sugar levels because your body digests it more slowly, this is according to researchers of a study published in 2008 in the *American Journal of Clinical Nutrition*. The American Diabetes Association agrees that the natural sugar in fruit does not pose a danger to diabetics because raw fruits have a low glycaemic index. Research in a small study concluded that people who ate twenty servings of fruit a day for twelve to twenty-four weeks suffered no ill effects. Diabetes UK also advises diabetics to eat fruit and vegetables since it reduces the risk of conditions such as high blood pressure, stroke, heart disease, obesity and some cancers – all of which diabetics are more susceptible to because of their condition.

Fruits and milk are packed with vitamins, minerals, protein and calcium besides the slow-release sugars, which is why they are not included in our daily guidelines for sugar consumption.

Sugar is addictive and eating it is a hard habit to break. Many of us have heard that sugar will boost flagging energy, but what you may not know is that it will actually cause an energy slump. Sugar fuels all the cells in our bodies, particularly our brain, which tells you sugar is a reward which only makes you want more. The more you eat sugar, the more you want. A sugar high, as it is known, occurs when a simple carbohydrate is turned into glucose in the bloodstream and causes a spike in blood sugar levels. When your body needs to move the glucose from the bloodstream and into the pancreas to make insulin, the energy levels drop leaving us shaky and tired. We then reach for the nearest sweet jar to maintain our sugar high. It is easily done, so it is easy to see why this can become a vicious cycle causing addictive habits set in. And, of course, any sugar not used up as energy by the body is stored as fat.

Sugars often go by a different name and you need to know these to be able to find them on food labels. These include:

Sucrose	Fructose	Glucose
Maltose	Dextrose	Lactose
Treacle	Honey	Golden syrup
Corn syrup	Maple syrup	Raw sugar
Inverted sugar syrup	Hydrolysed starch	

Its goes without saying that you pick the foods with the lowest amount of sugar and ditch the others – especially those sugary drinks which can contain up to nine teaspoons of sugar in each serving. As well as checking for sugars in the food label you can now identify sugar content by the traffic light system which is explained later, or with a smart phone app which you can download to scan products and discover how much sugar is in each one. Technology today can be really useful so try an app – it may just be the boost you need.

Salt

Salt is another massive problem as, like sugar, it is also hidden in most processed foods, in fact around 75 per cent of the salt we eat is already in ready-made foods such as bread, processed meats, soup and crisps. We are told regularly that too much salt is bad for us, but why? It comes down, once again, to heart disease, stroke, kidney disease and high blood pressure. The recommended daily intake of salt in this country is no more than 0.21oz (6g) daily, according to the World Health Organisation it should be no more than 0.17oz (5g) and yet the average person consumes around 0.28oz (8g). To ensure you are keeping track you can find the salt content on food labels and the salt content will be given per 3.5oz

(100g) serving. A high amount of salt would be more than 0.05oz (1.5g) per 3.5oz (100g) and a low amount is roughly 0.01oz (0.3g) per 3.5oz (100g). As salt is often hidden in processed foods there's a bit of guesswork involved but try to monitor as best you can by comparing different brands. The traffic light system explained later in the book will show you how to check if products are high in salt. You can reduce your salt intake by not using any when cooking or by cutting down. Keeping the salt-shaker on the table encourages us to consume more so hide it to avoid temptation at meal times. You can try low-salt food alternatives too and it's a good idea to cut down on ready meals and processed foods. We have been brought up to add salt to foods to stop them tasting bland, but if you swap salt for other flavourings such as black pepper, spices, herbs and even lemon juice, it'll not only be healthier for you but retrain your tastebuds to appreciate the real taste of foods.

Foods high in salt		
Bacon	Cheese	Gravy
Ham	Prawns	Salted Nuts
Bread	Pasta Sauces	Ready meals
Pizza	Soup	Sausages
Sauces		
Soy	Mayonnaise	Tomato ketchup

Fat

'If only mosquitoes sucked fat instead of blood.' Most people would love this to be true because the word 'fat' is so negative it automatically demotivates us. But what if I told you that there are fats that are beneficial? Yes, there really are. Let me explain. Since the body is unable to produce fatty acids independently, small amounts of some fats especially omega-3 are essential within our diets. In a nutshell, the fat you eat is made into fatty acids, which are smaller components of fat. These are used to create energy and are stored in the body's cells. If the fat is not used for this it then turns into body fat. There are two types of fat, saturated and unsaturated. The average man should consume no more than 1oz (30g) of fat a day and women no more than 0.7oz (20g). So what can we do? Swapping 'naughty' saturated fats for 'good' unsaturated fats can make a profound difference to a healthy lifestyle. Unsaturated fats are found in oil from plants believe it or not, and there are two types, monounsaturated, and polyunsaturated, which break down into omega-3 and omega-6. These healthy fats not only help manage your mood but also play a part in controlling your weight and fighting fatigue. So let us now look at the different fats, and the foods that contain them, and see if you can see why swapping these fats will make a difference.

High saturated fats	vs	Unsaturated fats
Fatty meats		Avocados
Sausages and pies		Nuts - almond, brazil, peanuts
Butter and Cream		Olive oil
Cheese - in particular hard cheese		Rapeseed oil
Good Fats		

Omega 3		
Oily fish	Kippers	Fresh tuna
Salmon	Sardines	Mackerel
Algae	Kale	Spinach

Omega 6	
Vegetable oil	Brazil nuts

Unsaturated fats are beneficial when it comes to reducing health risks. Omega 3 fats are essential fats that help in specific areas of health such as cognitive functioning and emotional health. Research has found that these Omega 3s and 6s can help:

Protect against memory loss and prevention of dementia
Reduce the risks of heart disease, stroke and cancer
Reduce the risk of and preventing ADHD, depression and bipolar disorder
Relieve joint pain and inflammatory skin conditions
Help with fatigue and stablising your mood
Help with pregnancy

In fact, not all fats are bad in the waistline wars, and the ways we can introduce more good fats into our diets are quite simple. For example, you could cook with olive oil or use it for dressing salads or vegetables; alternate it with flaxseed oil or extra virgin olive oil and avoid the ready-made salad dressings that are handy but extra-fattening. Avocados are super foods loaded with fats that are good for the brain and heart. They are versatile and can be added to salads or spread on sandwiches or toast. They are great with eggs. Snacking can be hard to give up so rather than reaching for chocolate, sweets or crisps, grab some nuts instead (no pun intended). Nuts can also be added to meals and are a great alternative to using breadcrumbs if cooking chicken or fish. You don't have to eliminate saturated fats completely, instead try these simple swaps which make a huge difference.

So let me put this all together for you. I know this information is a lot to take in, but it really is imperative to look at it closely as it will help you. To create a healthy diet, a person can take the information from food labels and calculate the energy, which is gained from the fat, protein and carbs. As we saw earlier:

> **1g of carbohydrates = 4 calories**
> **1g of protein = 4 calories**
> **1g of fat = 9 calories**

You can use this energy information to calculate the numbers of calories in a piece of food, or even in its breakdown of fat, protein and carbs. We will use a biscuit as an example;

If our biscuit's fat content is 3.2g, its protein 1.0g and its carbs 10.3g then you follow these calculations to work out the number of calories each of these contains

> **Calories from fat - 3.2 x 9 = 28 calories**
> **Calories from protein - 1.0 x 4= 4 calories**
> **Calories from carbs - 10.3 x 4 = 41.2 calories**

Try repeating this using a tin from your cupboard. If you struggle, just reread the bit above and all will become clear. You can combine this later in the chapter with an example of a meal plan.

Food Additivies

I will now briefly discuss food additives. Food additives are artificial or natural substances that are used within the manufacturing and processing of food and drink in order to prolong shelf life, add colour to our foods and add flavour or texture too. They have many functions in making our food safer and more appealing. EU legislation states that food additives must be declared on the packaging either through the additive's name or its E number. There are different types of common food additives: the first are antioxidants which stop food from decaying and discolouring particularly those which are prepared with fats or oils such as mayonnaise or soup mixes. The second is colouring which makes food look more attractive. Food can lose its natural colour when cooked or processed and so these are added to enhance the food's appearance and make it look brighter. Emulsifiers are added to ingredients such as oil and water to help them combine and stop them separating. Preservatives are added to food to keep them safely edible for longer by preventing growth of mould and fungus, they are often added to tinned food and cured or smoked meats. Some additives are natural such as beetroot juice, which is used as a colouring. Some are what's known as natural identical, which means they are chemically identical to natural flavourings but are man-made copies. Some vanilla flavourings fall into this category. Then there are artificial additives which are synthetically made and not a copy of natural substances. They add flavour, colour or sweetener to food and fizzy drinks. Finally, there are sweeteners – sugars which are added to foods to make them taste sweeter. Sweeteners are in fact low-calorie or calorie-free chemical ingredients and the most common are acesulfame K, aspartame, sorbitol, sucralose and saccharine. Saccharine, which is 300-400 times sweeter than sugar, was actually created in 1879 and was known as 'the poor man's sugar'. There have been claims over the years that sweeteners can increase people's chances of getting health conditions such as strokes, high blood pressure and cancer, however Cancer Research and the US National Cancer Institution have both said that there is no evidence for this. Sweeteners are also subjected to tests by the scientific committee of the European Food Safety Authority (EFSA) before any are used, to ensure they are safe and free from harm. So there are advantages and disadvantages to additives like any product. Let us take a look below at what these may be:

Advantages

- Food becomes more attractive from colouring
- Restores the colour of food and drink after the manufacturing process
- Food keeps its nutritional quality longer through preservation
- There is less waste as food will not be thrown away quickly
- Ingredients are not separated once they are combined when additives added
- Flavours can be enhanced
- Foods become more appealing once flavoured with additives
- Fish oils, vitamins and minerals can be added to food
- Additives can boost what is already naturally present in the food or can be artificially added

Disadvantages

- Since additives can be chemical substances created in a laboratory and there are still some concerns about how safe they are to consume
- Longterm risks aren't always known
- Children, particularly those with asthma or eczema, can develop allergies
- Additives can cause adverse reactions

The UK follows EU regulations on food additives. These are tested through the EFSA and each additive is given an E number. Up until 2015, there were 323 additives approved in the EU, 42 colours, 17 sweeteners, 36 preservatives, 18 anti-oxidants, 63 emulsions and 147 others. This may seem a lot to take in, but providing you with all this information will help you make informed decisions about the products you are purchasing.

Is this a lot of information to take in? Hopefully you are taking notes and you will have done the hard work calculating your BMI and BMR! We will be implementing all this further on but we need to know our nutritional needs firsts.

CHAPTER 3
NUTRITIONAL NEEDS OF INDIVIDUALS

'Take care of your body, it is the only place you live in'

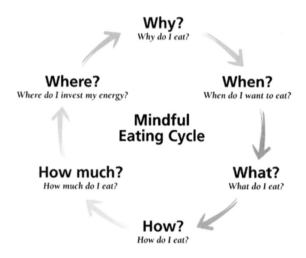

Tell me, who keeps us informed about what to eat and sets the daily recommendations? Because I get confused. First, we were told we should eat five pieces of fruit and veg a day, then the professionals were saying it should be seven a day and the last I heard it was twelve a day! There are endless headlines telling us fruit and veg prevent obesity, heart disease, strokes and diabetes, etc., or that we should or shouldn't eat red meat, or drink red wine. It would be nice to know, in simple terms, what the general benefits are and how they affect the human body and our health. So I will discuss this here as I think it is pretty important. If you do not know the advantages of the foods you are eating, what gives you the incentive to eat healthily?

Eating healthily is as much about eating the right food as it is about how much you're consuming. If you can get the perfect balance of the foods, you're good to go. We will look now at what it is recommended our plates should contain and what the advantages of each element are.

The Eatwell Plate

This plate has been divided in to sections to show us the proportions of each food group we should be consuming every day. It doesn't need to balance out precisely every day, but should even out over a week. Fruit and vegetables and carbohydrates should each make up over a third of your daily intake. Of the remaining quarter, proteins take up just over half, dairy just under half and the rest a tiny sliver is unsaturated fats. Sugary snacks, sweets, alcohol and crisps don't feature on the Eatwell Plate at all and should be kept to occasional treats. In addition to this you should drink six to eight glasses of water a day.

Carbohydrates and sugars

People think carbohydrates are bad for you, but actually they are an important part of our diet as they provide energy. In fact, low-carb diets can actually make people ill if they are taken to extremes. Carbs should make up 33 per cent of our daily diet, however people who are physically active should get more of their calories from carbs and there are two types. Simple carbs, which are found in milk, fruit and vegetables, they are natural sugars which are converted by the body into energy. Don't go confusing these natural sugars with the refined sugars in cakes and biscuits and sweets – these might provide energy but they lack vitamins and fibre and are also high in fat. Complex carbs, which are starches and fibres and come from foods such as rice, pasta and potatoes. They release energy more slowly, aid digestion and guard against type 2 diabetes and heart disease. They are your friends when it comes to weight-loss as they keep you feeling full for longer. Refined sugar should only make up 1 per cent of our daily diet since it has no nutritional benefit. However, as we tend to favour sugary fattening foods over more nutritional foods this leads to weight gain. Sugary foods are less filling than starchy foods, which is why you become hungry quicker after eating them. Starchy carbs are better at stabilising your blood sugar and your energy levels and these are found in wholegrains. Wholegrain or wholemeal bread is more beneficial as is wholemeal pasta, quinoa, brown rice and porridge oats. We spoke about sugars in the previous chapter; fructose is a natural sugar found in fruit and is healthier than the refined sugar which you add to tea and coffee.

Protein

Protein is our next source. We need protein for energy, body growth and repairing blood cells. When we eat protein it is broken down by the digestive system into amino acids, which are then absorbed and used by our body to make new proteins. Protein has many purposes such as building muscle tissue, improving the quality of our skin, hair and fingernails and making the anti-bodies which boost immunity.

Protein makes up 15 per cent of our diet. How much protein we need depends on our gender and age. Take a look below:

	Age	Protein (g per day)
Men	19-50	56
	50+	53
Women	19-50	45
	50+	47

Meats are high in protein so chicken, pork and turkey are good sources, as are fish, which is full of omega fats, eggs and dairy products such as low-fat milk. If you are a vegetarian then you will need to find your protein from other sources such as beans, lentils, pulses and Quorn.

Both animal protein and vegetable protein have their advantages and disadvantages. Animal has higher biological value, which simply means that it is easier for the body to use. Vegetable protein sources have a lower biological value so they are harder for the body to use, but on the plus side they lack saturated fat and contain fibre. You need to minimise saturated fats from animal sources. This can be done simply by avoiding processed foods such as sausages, burgers, salami, pork pies, and breaded meat such as chicken nuggets and chicken kiev. Other tips to consider are removing skin from meat and cutting off the fat.

To ensure you get the maximum benefit from protein, I would advise choosing widely from both kinds.

Milk and dairy

Milk and dairy products make up 8 per cent of our diet that is to two to three portions a day. Milk is not only full of calcium, which we need for strong and healthy bones but it also gives us protein. Semi-skimmed milk is the most popular milk in the UK. If you want more calcium with fewer calories and fat, then skimmed milk is the better option so make a simple swap. In addition to milk, there is yogurt, cream and cheese.

Cream is high in fat and the thicker it is the more fat it contains, which is why you should always look for healthy alternatives. Be mindful of the 'low-fat' cream as it may contain high sugar levels. Yogurts, if not chocolate or the sweet kind, can be beneficial as they can give the protein we need. Try fat-free yogurt, live or natural yogurt as a healthier option.

Water

Is water as important as the professionals say it is? YES, it is! It is essential and, though you could go without food for several weeks, without water we would only survive a few days. Did you know that our body weight is around two thirds water? Our recommended water intake is six to eight glasses per day. Tea, coffee and juice all count towards your fluid intake and, technically, so do fizzy drinks, however I don't recommend them as they are high in sugar and calories but don't offer any nutritional benefit. You are probably now thinking does alcohol count? No, unfortunately it does not, for a whole variety of reasons but I'll be discussing alcohol and calories later on. If you think pure water is too plain and you just cannot drink it (I know many people feel like this), I have written a specific section just for you further on so you won't miss out.

Why do we need water?

Without water our bodies just would not function. An important factor to remember is we lose water through sweating and when we use the toilet. How many times a day do you nip to the loo for a pee? Think of how much you are losing then. That's why we stress the importance of drinking water. Here are some other reasons:

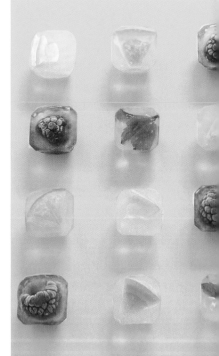

- **Our body needs water to control its temperature to cool down when hot, this is done through sweating**

- **Water removes toxic waste from your body**

- **Our joints need protecting and water does this job. If you don't drink enough water your muscles become stiff**

- **It protects our brain and spinal cord as it acts as a shock absorber**

- **Helps with the digestive process**

- **Metabolises our food**

- **Keeps us hydrated**

- **Helps keep our skin look younger**

- **Energises our muscles**

- **Helps us go the toilet**

Beat the bloat

To beat the bloat, you need to follow all the advice in this book from healthy eating, to drinking water. Feeling bloated can leave our stomachs feeling fat and uncomfortable. The most common reasons for this are constipation, periods and conditions such as IBS, coeliac disease and food intolerance.

Cut out fizzy drinks, processed and sugary foods, which cause wind. Increase your potassium levels by eating foods such as bananas, asparagus, melon, citrus fruits and tomatoes, which can help relieve your stomach from bloating. Drinking water will help flush out any nasty toxins within the stomach and gut area. Exercise helps with this too so build some into your regime since it promotes bowel movement. Women can suffer with bloating during the 'time of the month'. Try massaging your stomach to help with the pains and bloating or take herbal remedies such as primrose oil, which have been proven to help. Your diet is an important factor in any bloating and therefore you should eat healthily, stick to low-sodium foods and cut out the bread, which can add to the problem. If you have a medical condition that leads to bloating, you should speak to your GP about ways to reduce it as they may have alternatives for you to try.

The benefits of drinking water are endless but the consequences from not drinking any fluids and from becoming dehydrated can be catastrophic. You can also get water from eating fruits and vegetables so stock up on these and don't forget to keep a bottle of water in your car or at home to keep your body functioning correctly. Speaking of fruits and veggies, we will now move on to the next nutrients our body needs which are contained in these.

Vitamins and minerals

Micronutrients are another name for vitamins and minerals because we only need them in minute quantities. They help with the production of hormones and support our immune system against any harmful substances and germs, therefore they act as a defender of the body. They also control body processes and set off chemical reactions, which are necessary to our bodily functions. Without the minerals our bodies would fall to pieces. If you do not receive these micronutrients you will find yourself with one of two types of deficiencies; primary or secondary. Primary deficiencies occur when you don't have enough vitamins and minerals in your diet and secondary deficiencies occur when you are not absorbing enough from your diet, which can be due to old age, smoking, alcohol problems or medical conditions.

Minerals are obtained from eating plants and animals and the major minerals are iron, calcium, magnesium and phosphorous. All have extremely important functions from production of healthy blood cells to building health bones and a healthy nervous system. Vitamins are stored within our body fat, meaning we can access them easily if our body is not getting enough from our diet. It will be discussed in a later chapter how this can be dangerous for those who consume vitamin supplements, but first let me explain the types of vitamins and what they do.

Vitamin A is a fat-soluble vitamin. It is needed to maintain good eyesight, especially night vision. Vitamin A deficiency can lead to night blindness. It is also needed for healthy skin and mucous membranes as well as strong immunity against infection. People who are at risk of deficiencies are those with medical conditions, which make it difficult to absorb fats. Green vegetables are a great source of Vitamin A, as are mackerel and milk.

Vitamin D is also a fat-soluble vitamin, and we can make it in our bodies through a chemical reaction when our skin is exposed to sunlight. We need this type of vitamin to maintain healthy bones and teeth, as it helps the body to absorb and use calcium. People at risk from lack of vitamin D are those who are confined indoors or people who remain covered up by clothes. The risk of not getting enough of this vitamin can cause rickets and pain in our bones and joints. The best dietary sources are from oily fish, eggs, meat and dairy products and, of course, sunlight.

Vitamin E is another fat-soluble vitamin. It is needed in our immune systems and our reproductive systems as well as being an important antioxidant needed for cell protection, particularly in those with medical conditions who may lack vitamin E. Avocado, spinach, nuts and seeds are the best sources.

Vitamin K is produced naturally within our gut by harmless bacteria, and is a fat-soluble vitamin needed to help our bones remain healthy and our blood to clot. People who require antibiotics for long periods of time often lack vitamin K because the medication has killed off the bacteria. Sources include asparagus, leafy greens, eggs and fish oils.

Vitamin C is a water-soluble vitamin, the best-known form of which is ascorbic acid. We need it to heal wounds and maintain healthy connective tissues. It helps with a healthy immune system and also helps our body absorb iron from food. Those at risk of deficiency are smokers and people who do not eat enough fruit and vegetables. Deficiency in vitamin C can lead to scurvy, muscle pain and tiredness. We get vitamin C from citrus fruits such as lemons as well as sprouts, broccoli and tomatoes. But the fruit most famously associated with vitamin C is the orange. Many people think of vitamin C and connect this to an orange automatically. Don't forget the other sources too!

There are a variety of B vitamins which are also water-soluble vitamins, let's take a look at their properties and health benefits:

Vitamin B1 releases energy from food. People who abuse alcohol and drugs are at risk of lacking this, which we can obtain from pork, nuts and seeds.

Vitamin B2 fights stress and helps us digest proteins and carbs. Some medical conditions cause deficiency as the patient can't fully absorb the vitamin. Our best way to obtain B2 is from consuming meat, eggs, watercress and spinach.

The next B vitamin is B3, which releases energy from our food and helps keep our skin and nervous system healthy. We can get this from wheatflour, peas, meat and dairy products. Those at risk of deficiency are women who take oral contraceptives and smokers.

Vitamin B6 helps control our moods and helps our bodies store energy from protein and carbohydrates. It also helps form haemoglobin, the substance in red blood cells that carries oxygen round the body. Again smokers and people who abuse alcohol are most at risk of being deficient. To avoid risking a deficiency in this vitamin then consume pork, chicken, eggs and beans along with potatoes and brown rice.

Folic acid is another B vitamin and, as we all know, pregnant woman and women trying to conceive are advised to take this to help ensure their foetus develops healthily. The rest of us need folic acid for our immune system and to help our bodies absorb nutrients effectively. To ensure we get our folic acid intake we should eat eggs, green veggies, citrus fruits and broccoli. Those who may be at risk of not receiving sufficient folic acid are the elderly, pregnant women and those who do not eat enough vegetables.

Lastly, B12 is used for the production of red blood cells and for processing folic acid. Sources of B12 are red meat (in moderation), salmon, cod, yeast extract and eggs. Vegetarians and vegans are most at risk from not consuming enough vitamin B12.

Minerals are vital for health. Some minerals you may have heard of include calcium, iron, magnesium and phosphorus.

Let us start with calcium, which is associated with healthy bones and teeth but also important for muscle function and blood clotting. Milk and dairy products are a good source of calcium, as is fish (fresh or tinned), tofu, figs, kale and almonds.

Next is iron, though not many people are aware this is a mineral. We need it to produce haemoglobin in our red blood cells in order to carry oxygen around the body and to stop us getting conditions such as anaemia. Vegetarians and women who have heavy periods are at risk of having a deficiency and the best source is from meat: liver being the best, but also red meat and chicken. Pulses are a source as are nuts and dried fruits.

Magnesium is needed for healthy bones and muscle function and also to help our bodies deal with stress and we can consume meat, green veggies and mushrooms to ensure we don't miss out.

The main function of phosphorus is to make healthy bones and teeth but it also supports a healthy functioning nervous system. It is found in most foods, animal and veggie sources.

Trace Elements

Trace elements, which include zinc, copper, selenium, iodine and chromium, are also essential to a healthy diet.

Zinc is important for preventing infection and for sperm production. The best sources are from shellfish, oysters, meat and green leafy veggies.

Copper is needed for healthy blood vessels, nerves and bones. Meat, seafood, wholemeal bread, green veggies, nuts and seeds are all sources from which we can receive our copper intake.

Selenium helps protect against heart disease and cancer, so people who smoke are at risk of not getting enough of this mineral. We can find this in meat, Brazil nuts, seafood and eggs.

Iodine is used to make thyroid hormones and it is found in spinach, red meat and egg yolks.

Finally, chromium which, alongside insulin, regulates our blood sugar level. We find it in lean red meat, potatoes, eggs, apples and broccoli.

The best sources of vitamins and mineral are, of course, fruit and vegetables, which should make up 33 per cent of our diet or the equivalent of five portions daily. We know fruit and veg are full of vitamins and minerals and also contain fibre. You can actually include fruit and veggies that are fresh, frozen or tinned as part of your daily intake. Most people think that potatoes are classed as vegetables but they are in fact grouped as carbohydrates because of their high starch content. Adding potatoes is probably the best change you can make to your diet as they will help with your digestive system and they are full of nutrients while being low in calories.

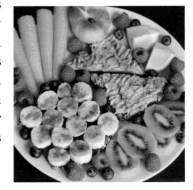

Fibre

Another good thing about potatoes is that they contain fibre. Dietary fibre is the material in food that cannot be digested, in particular, cellulose from plant cell walls. Fibre is an important part of the diet, it keeps food moving efficiently through the digestive system and helps keep our blood sugars balanced. It is also great for our dental health too as it helps saliva flow. According to statistics most people in the UK get about 18g of fibre a day when we should be aiming for at least 30g a day. There are three types of fibre; insoluble, soluble and resistant starch.

Insoluble fibre helps prevent diarrhoea and constipation, the best type of sources are veggies and fruits, wholegrains and nuts.

Soluble fibre helps lower blood cholesterol and slows down the rate at which glucose is absorbed into the bloodstream. The best sources of this type of fibre are oats, fruit, peas, beans, lentils and seeds.

Resistant starch cannot be broken down by digestive enzymes and so it passes into the large intestine where it helps bacteria within the bowel and helps us absorb vitamins and minerals. The best sources of this are wholegrains, beans and lentils. So fibre-rich foods are vegetables, fruits and wholegrains and since fibre is a main constituent of our diet, look for foods with a high fibre intake when shopping – it'll tell you on the label. Fibre can help with weight-loss since it makes food more satisfying helping us feeling fuller for longer and resistant to the urge to snack between meals.

Glycaemic index

The glycaemic index (GI) basically describes the rise in blood sugar that results from eating a given food. A food with a high GI will produce a short rapid increase in our blood sugars while foods with a low GI produce smaller changes and a longer-lasting effect. To sustain energy, we want low-GI foods. If you eat out a lot, eat highly-processed foods or white foods such as processed pasta and bread then you will be eating high GI foods. Foods with low GI are the usual veggies, fruits, wholemeal or wholegrain, beans and lentils. You need a rough idea of how the GI works as you may come across it but choosing which foods to eat if you do is quite logical.

So we have discussed the components for a healthy diet but let us take a look at some key words that you may have heard of and also new words, which have suddenly popped up in the latest health trends.

Clean eating

This has become popular over the last few years and you may have read about it in a magazine or seen it promoted on supermarket shelves. So what is clean eating? If you typed this into a search engine on the internet, you would get a variety of different answers, in actual fact from one particular search engine there were roughly 27,200,000 results. Always look for a trusted source, such as the NHS website, when looking for an answer or it will be confusing or even misleading.

Clean eating is basically just eating a healthy and balanced diet full of nutritious foods and avoiding processed and refined foods. We know this already, but introducing new terms can make people want to follow the 'trend'. Keep it simple or you will over-complicate things. Clean eating is everything this book is about.

Phytochemicals

Simply a variety of compounds produced by plants. The word 'phyto' means plant in Greek and so the meaning is 'plant chemicals'. Certain phytochemicals can act as antioxidants while others may be beneficial for our blood lipid levels. Vegetables contain vitamins that are phytochemicals and others that are pigments making cabbages green and carrots orange. They are also the chemicals which give onions their smell. Some examples of phytochemicals are:

Allicin – Antioxidants from onions and garlic, which can help protect our cells from free radicals within the body

Flavonoids – Antioxidants that can be found in apple skins, grapes and olives

Lutein – Found in vegetables, particularly green leafy types and orange and yellow fruits. It is important for eye health.

There are many phytochemicals and their benefits in fruit and vegetables are myriad. There are many studies being conducted to show how powerful they are and their positive effects in human health.

Antioxidants – This word crops up today in every health article, newspaper, medical study, diet trend and even on social media. So what are antioxidants and why are they good for us? Antioxidants protect our cells by reacting with free radicals before they cause oxidative damage. They either prevent cell damage altogether or delay the effects. Antioxidants are available as dietary supplements, however it is advised that you get your antioxidants from food. This is not to say supplements do not work: as long as they are backed by science and research then you should be fine. For example, supplements which contain fruit or vegetable extracts may be beneficial to you. Some of the best foods to

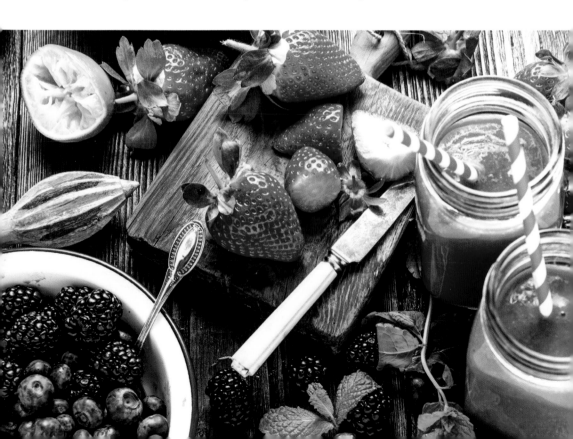

get antioxidants from are prunes, blueberries, strawberries, oranges, raspberries, red grapes, kale, sprouts, red peppers, onions and spinach.

Free radicals

Free radicals damage our body's cells. They are produced naturally so are hard to avoid, which is why consuming antioxidants helps protect us. Examples of free radicals are cigarette smoke, burnt food, sun exposure and pollution, which in turn might lead to health problems such as heart disease, strokes, Alzheimer's disease and cancer. Berries are a good source of antioxidants as they can help the ageing process too. Speaking of berries, we will now look at the theory about colours of foods and how counting colours may benefit us.

What is the colour of your diet?

Have you ever heard people say you should 'eat the rainbow'? This is because they believe that, instead of counting calories, you should load your plate with colourful vegetables and fruits as different coloured foods bring different health benefits. I don't see the point in this since as fruits and veggies are low in calories anyway, however, colours can brighten our mood so let us brighten our diets too. The brighter the better. I will discuss 'super foods' later, but for now let us look at the colours of food and their effects.

Orange and yellow sources –
Orange, clementine, nectarine, lemon, banana, pineapple, pumpkin, sweet potato

White sources –
Onion, cauliflower, mushroom, garlic, cabbage

Red sources –
Strawberries, cherries, watermelon, cranberries, raspberries, apple, grapes

Blue and purple sources –
Blueberries, blackberries, plum, red onion, aubergine

Green sources –
Broccoli, kiwi, kale, lettuce, cabbage, apple, grapes, avocado, spinach, pear, lime

Not only are all these bright and beautiful colours but they are also full of phytonutrients, vitamins, minerals and also fibre. This picture shows how appetising your diet could be and, to me, it looks much more appealing than a bar of chocolate or fizzy drink. Colourful food is also more attractive and since we eat first with our eyes, a colourful plate is more likely to stimulate our appetites.

The way we eat our food

The way we eat our food can be seen as a factor in our weight gain or loss. In France, workers take long lunch breaks and because they eat slowly, they digest slowly, probably enjoying it more and feeling fuller at the end. If you eat quickly you are often hungry a few hours later. Studies have shown that eating a healthy meal gives you a feeling of satisfaction and fullness so you do not feel you need to snack later on. The problem with our society is that everyone rushes their food or skips meals. For example, people who do not eat breakfast often feel the urge to snack by mid-morning, they eat again at lunchtime, then have an energy slump in the afternoon and end up snacking all day. Those who eat ready meals or rubbish food find themselves hungrier due to a sugar crash and need more sugar to maintain their blood and sugar levels. People need to look at the bigger picture and realise that if you eat three proper meals a day you will feel the need to snack less and if you do snack then you will feel like snacking on healthier food.

Eating as a family is also a great way to sit and concentrate on your food. Meals become a celebration of family as well as of eating. Food becomes a nourishment instead of an inconvenience to be fitted into a busy day.

The saying 'breakfast is the most important meal of the day' is true. Breakfast gives us that energy boost we need after a good night sleep and sets us up for

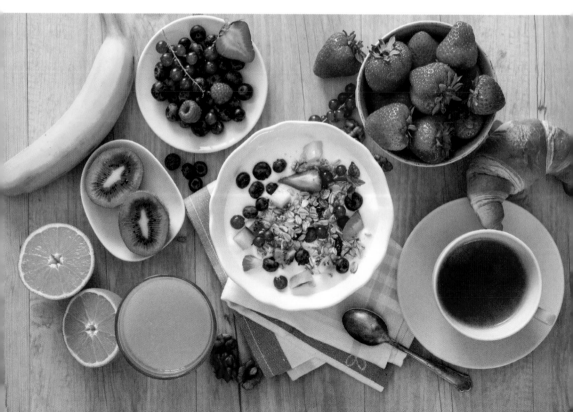

the day ahead. Studies have shown one in four of us skip breakfast. I used to do the same in my previous job as a care worker. Long shifts and stress made it hard and often left me feeling weak in the afternoon or evenings. Often I'd resort to chocolates and crisps for an energy boost to see me through the remainder of my shift. It is easily done I know but, by taking ten minutes out to eat breakfast, you are sustaining your energy levels for the whole of the day and avoiding the cravings that could plague you. Waking up ten minutes earlier to consume breakfast is not a big factor – when you see this written down it looks simple, but will be massively effective for you.

Before you eat determine whether you are making the right food choices.

Ask yourself these four questions. The immediate response you receive is your subconscious telling you the true answer:

Will this food leave me feeling full of energy or feeling drained?
Will this food make me feel amazing or bad about myself?
Will this food destroy my body in the long run or will it nourish it?
Will eating this food show respect or contempt for not only my body but also my mind?

Researchers have completed studies about how we think about our food. It is called 'mindful eating'. In the *Harvard Health Letter*, published by the Harvard Medical School, the author says: 'Applied to eating, mindfulness includes noticing the colours, smells, flavours, and textures of your food; chewing slowly; getting rid of distractions like TV or reading; and learning to cope with guilt and anxiety about food. Some elements of mindful eating hark back to Horace Fletcher, an early twentieth-century food faddist, known as The Great Masticator, who believed chewing food thoroughly would solve many different kinds of health problems.

This is the way to change our lifestyles for the better by enjoying everything about the process. If you change your thoughts about your body and lifestyle, then you will change how your body looks.

Now we have spoken about the principles of healthy eating, we need to look at physical exercise. If you hate exercise, then this section may help you understand more why it is so important. So many people hate exercise but there are so many activities you can engage in which are fun rather than boring. If you need motivation to do exercise then ask a friend or family member to do it with you or even hire a personal trainer or go to a class. These sessions might cost but they work, as long as you stick it out and attend every week! Remember YOU are in control!'

Physical exercise – do we need to do it?

Is it necessary to do exercise? People who diet often think that they do not need to do any physical exercise. Turning your life round to lose weight is a massive achievement but good health does not happen overnight and everyone needs exercise in line with weight-loss diets. Why? For medical reasons, to keep us active, to stop us becoming overweight, to keep our bodies functioning correctly. If you are not an active person then start slowly rather than jumping into physical exercise, struggling and then giving up. This is where planning your regimes will help.

Physical exercise is not just about losing weight, getting fit and toning up. It has so many more advantages. 'If exercise were a pill, it would be one of the most cost-effective drugs ever invented,' says Dr Nick Cavill, a research associate of the University of Oxford. This is because it helps, not only with the prevention of health conditions such as strokes, obesity, type 2 diabetes and cancer, but it can also help beat stress and depression, boost self-esteem and even put you in a better mood. So why don't we do it?

A big reason is due to convenience and technology. Before cars were invented or before people had jobs how did they get to work? They walked and they cycled now we just jump in the car, on the bus or train or in a taxi to get us to the places we need to go. We also have the luxury of labour-saving devices such as washing machines, dryers and irons, which take the strain out of domestic life. Sounds so simple but it is so true. If you are a builder or roofer you do strenuous work and will have good activity levels. But studies have shown that today many people sit down at computer screens for their job, not for a couple of hours but for seven at a time. What did we do before computers? What about our hobbies? How many people leave work and go for a run or how many go home and sit on their phones, computers or laptops and watch the TV? Previous generations were more active through work and necessity and the point I am trying to get across is that if you simply added more activity levels to your daily life this would have a significant improvement on your health and waistline!

So what if you chose to walk to the shops or work rather than driving? If you walked thirty minutes each way, this could add on an hour of physical activity per day. Rather than taking the children or grandchildren to the local indoor play area, how about a walk around the park or to a local beach? That could add an extra two hours to your daily activity level. In many cities now they have bikes for hire funded by local councils and it has become a big trend to use them for days out or sight-seeing. It is a fun way to exercise and it's nice to see the pictures all over social media. And for would-be runners there are downloadable Couch to 5K running programmes to get you out into the fresh air. There are recommendations for exercises and levels of intensity to suit everyone, but I believe you need to choose one you enjoy and you can manage. There are so many classes available now – even men- or women-only classes (if you're feeling a bit shy) and over-sixty-five classes. A new one on the scene called Glow fit is a dance rave where everyone exercises! How great is that? I am sure you would love it. Yoga and meditation are always popular: not only are you exercising but also clearing your mind too, and there are Zumba and dance classes. These are just a few ideas of ways you can introduce some exercise into your daily routine. Plan on increasing activity levels week after week, once you see results from any form of exercise, it becomes addictive.

Having an inactive lifestyle has more disadvantages than you would know: It is described by the Department of Health as the 'silent killer' because people who sit or lie around are more likely to suffer with bad health. This is why exercise is important. Two and a half hours of moderate exercise a week is the level you should aim for if you are fit and well. Forms of moderate exercise include walking fast, hiking or even using a lawn mower and cutting the grass. This will raise your heart rate and make you breathe faster so you should be able to talk but can't sing the words to a song. The idea of vigorous exercise puts people off even starting any form of exercise but this is the level you are aiming to get to if you aren't already there. It includes playing football, rugby or tennis, running, cycling and swimming. This may sound daunting, and you need to introduce this exercise in small amounts to know what you are aiming for in the long run. If you start with an hour's workout after not exercising for years you will have sore muscles, be exhausted and probably filled with dread about completing another exercise routine. If you are not used to doing exercise or have a medical condition, particularly a heart condition, you should talk to your doctor before starting any routines. He or she will probably be able to suggest some ways you can safely build up your stamina.

Look at some of these activities, some of which we do daily, and the calories we can lose just by completing them:

Activity	Calories used in 30 minutes
Ironing	69 calories
Cleaning & dusting	75 calories
Walking	99 calories
Cleaning with a vacuum	105 calories
Golf	129 calories
Brisk walking	150 calories
Running (10 mins to a mile)	300 calories

When you look at these, imagine how many calories you could burn by adding in another exercise. Look at these numbers and set some goals of how many minutes exercise you would like to complete.

Benefits of exercising

There are numerous benefits to exercising apart from just losing weight and maintaining weight-loss. As I have mentioned before there is lots of medical evidence to show it can reduce the risk of major illnesses. It can lower your risk of coronary heart disease and stroke by 35 per cent, your risk of type 2 diabetes by 50 per cent and your risk of early death by 30 per cent

Exercise is known to improve your mood, which helps if you suffer with depression, anxiety or stress. It is calculated that exercise lowers the risk of depression by 30 per cent. It does this is by stimulating brain chemicals known as endorphins. Endorphins interact with receptors in our brain and leave us feeling happier and more relaxed. This helps with self-confidence and self-esteem and makes us feel better about our appearance. As well as boosting our mood it boosts our energy and improves our muscle strength by helping our cardiovascular system work more efficiently, giving us more energy, improving our posture, lowering our cholesterol and strengthening our bones.

If you struggle with starting exercise, then meet with a fitness coach who will be able to talk you through the activities which will suit you best or which classes you might enjoy. You may even have a local walking or running club you could join and if you are feeling really brave why not try some boxing. Many men play five-a-side football, which is great for your fitness levels. If you are a bit shy about exercising in front of other people, then you could do your own home workouts from a DVD or even the internet. The options are endless, however only you can decide whether you want to embark on this journey.

If there is a barrier to you exercising speak to your local council about what they may offer for those with medical conditions or disabilities. For example, swimming baths and leisure centres often offer alternative activities for individuals who struggle.

Don't forget you don't need to consult a GP or medical professional about exercise, unless you have a pre-existing condition or are concerned about your health. It is free, easy to find and it has immediate effects.

Another benefit of exercising is that it improves sleeping patterns, especially if you suffer with insomnia, but then sleeping is a big part of weight-loss too. Let's see why.

Sleep

When you become tired you reach for something that will perk you up. I always found chocolate worked, but others may reach for a sugary drink, energy drink or of course coffee. It's natural that we become tired, but it can also be a vicious cycle that we can become stuck in. You feel tired mid-afternoon, you reach for comfort food, you skip your exercise after work and because you can't be bothered to cook you throw a ready meal in the microwave or order a takeaway. I know – I have been there. Sleep deprivation can cause weight gain and damage your health too. I am not saying sleep all the time and you will lose weight, but not having enough sleep can mean your metabolism doesn't work in the right way. However, if you have a good night's sleep, how much more energetic do you feel the next day? It's recommended we have seven hours a night, but people who work shifts or have newborn babies will struggle with this. If you are having trouble sleeping, think about what you are doing before you go to bed. For example, having caffeine before you sleep is not the best idea, neither is eating a burger or pizza as not only will the calories sit on you, so will heartburn, which is most definitely going to keep you up through the night. Look at your sleep pattern to see if there are any changes you could make to ensure you have an undisturbed sleep. Not only will good sleep stop you reaching for the comfort or energy food, it will also help you if you are stressed or anxious. Swapping your bad bedtime foods for healthy ones will curb your cravings and keep you full until breakfast.

Nobody likes a grouch and with so many benefits of having a decent night's sleep, you should make sure you are receiving the correct amount each night. That way you'll function properly and stay focused: studies have shown that sleep increases brain agility, memory and creativity. Just imagine the amount you could get done with a good night's sleep.

I would like us to think about our bodies and food before we start developing a guide which suits you. Remember this about changing our thoughts about food and drink and all the different elements to go with it. See it as a jigsaw and we are putting all the pieces together.

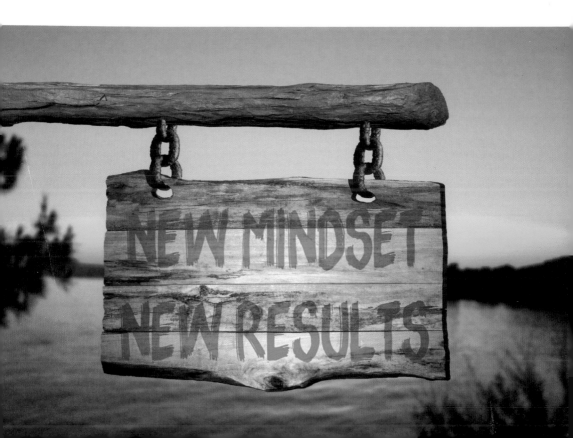

CHAPTER 4

WHY DO WE EAT AND HOW TO OVERCOME THIS

'Be the best version of YOU'

Why do we overeat?

There are a variety of reasons why we overeat. Take a look at the subjects below and see if you can identify with any of them:

Boredom	Routine
Emotional eating	Anxiety
Upset	Hormones
Habit	How you were brought up
Stress	Occasions
Social	Binge eating
Stopping smoking	Medical
Pressure	Energy
Addicted to sugars	Readily Available
Just because food's there	

As you can see, it's not just because we are hungry. Many of you will probably be able to identify with at least one of the reasons above as our emotions, habits and routines play a big part in our everyday lives. Eating without thinking can hurt our weight goals. Let us try and figure out some ways in which you can adapt to overcome these obstacles.

Binge eating disorder (BED) is the most serious as it can lead to obesity. Binge eating disorder is when someone eats large quantities of food in a short amount of time and has no control over their diet. People often yo-yo between this and dieting and the vicious circle it creates is hard to control. The short-term effect of BED is general physical discomfort, but it can lead to obesity when sugar cravings become uncontrollable. This occurs when rising and falling blood sugar levels send false messages to the brain giving you cravings for food your body does not actually need. This in turn can lead to emotional problems such as anxiety and depression, low self-esteem and lack of confidence, which in turn can cause life traumas such as loneliness. Long-term effects from BED are asthma and back pain, sleep apnoea, cancer, heart disease, heart failure and even strokes. All these conditions are caused by not eating a healthy balanced diet and consuming too much sugar and fatty food which the body is unable to break down.

Emotional eating is a form of trigger. We eat in celebration when we are happy; we eat when we are sad because food is comforting; we eat when we are angry because it suppresses the emotion; we eat when we are under pressure as a coping technique and we eat when we are stressed as we often have no other strategy in place to turn to.

If you could have a mechanism in place to help you control your feelings, then you would be able to identify what works for YOU! I used to eat when I was bored or hormonal so I put a plan in place so I could tackle this head on. I wrote down a list of things I enjoyed – fun alternatives to occupy my body and my mind. My list consisted of simple things such as going for a walk, calling a friend or family member, put on a DVD, even brushing my teeth. Once you are past that first craving of food it's over. You could even try writing a diary: when you feel like eating, write your thoughts down. Not only does this clear your mind but putting a pen to paper is a proven release mechanism. You need to recognise your own hunger levels to be able to tell whether you really are hungry or just being greedy, something we are all guilty of at times!

Stress is an unavoidable part of modern life. It can be challenging because not only do we suppress it by comfort eating but it can also lead to other health problems such as insomnia, skin problems, migraines, constipation and IBS. We overeat when stressed, particularly on junk food, so we need to swap this habit for one of good nutrition. One simple idea to cut down on ready meals is to prepare meals in advance and store them in the freezer. Cooking frozen vegetables and nice piece of fish is better than phoning for a takeaway and takes less time than it does for your meal to be delivered. Prepping salads one night for the rest of the week is also a convenient way of avoiding ready meals. Fresh soups are quick and easy to make and great to have in stock. Instead of sweets and crisps, keep a supply of healthy snacks rich in vitamin C to hand. Vitamin C levels decrease when we are stressed and since vitamin C cannot be stored in the body you should always have citrus fruits or strawberries available to snack on. Many stressful situations can be out of your control, but if you manage the parts of the situation you can control with pre-planned coping mechanisms such as meditation or reading a book, you will be able to deal with the stress better – and without reaching for a sugar boost. YOU are in control, not the food.

Eating out can be another obstacle to healthy eating. Enjoying time with family and friends is great, but are you one of those people who eats out for the sake of it? Research has shown that our habits imitate our companion's actions in situations like these and we can find ourselves eating more simply because our companion is. This is especially true at buffets where the food looks too scrumptious, the cakes too divine and the cocktails even better. Think of it this way: you are there to mingle, so focus on the conversation or the person who is celebrating a special occasion. Either skip the food or take your own low-calorie treat. You may be thinking I only go to a party once a year, in which case don't worry about it too much. This is for those of you who eat out or attend a social events regularly, for example as part of your job.

When food is just there in plain sight, it is easy to grab and eat it. And many of us would think where is the harm? Add up how many times you do this a week including during meal preparation and shopping, which is discussed later. We all need some willpower to resist temptation. Put a photo on the fridge or cupboard door so you will see it before you reach for a snack. This may be a picture of the 'new you' or a dress you'd like to wear. Even better remove any temptations and treats before you start your lifestyle change. If you don't eat a healthy and balanced diet, you will probably experience a slump in the middle of the afternoon. For an energy boost you'll probably pop to the shop or vending machine for a bar of chocolate. But a sugary snack always equals a sugar crash so ensure you have a healthy snack such as a banana to hand instead – it will help you beat that slump.

Are you one of these people who eats at the same time every day? Sometimes routines such as work commitments or children's meals dictate when we eat. But just because the clock says it's dinner time does not mean we are actually hungry. This kind of eating is a habit, so check your hunger levels and prepare your meal accordingly.

Do you feel the need to please people all the time? Often when we visit family and friends we accept a drink and maybe a cake because we don't want to offend them. Having an excuse ready beforehand will make it easier to say no. You don't need to explain yourself, just politely say no thank you and don't be pushed into eating something when you don't feel like it. You are in control.

Are you a person who always clears the plate? When you were growing up how many times did you hear your parents say 'there are people who would be grateful for that food,' resulting in guilty eating! Have you ever cleared your plate even though you felt full and then felt sick? A way around this is simple: portion control. Only put on your plate what you know you can manage; even buy smaller plates or use the pattern on the plate to measure portion control.

If you feel you have a serious issue with food, then get in touch with a medical profession such as your GP or a reliable support group who will be able to help and guide you in the way that you need.

No matter what you are feeling, always remember that it is YOU and only YOU that is in control. Food is an addiction so have these plans, lists and pictures in place ready to beat your demons. If you can say no, then you are half way there. The next part of the chapter is about positivity and body image which will help build your confidence now we have learnt how to tackle the addiction.

Principles of Weight Management

Have you ever read a magazine article or glanced at a picture, scrolled through social media or looked at the TV and thought 'I wish I looked like that' or 'I want a toned stomach like that?' Maybe even 'I wish I had that person's healthy way of life and motivation?' Well, you are not alone and these are all part of the thought patterns associated with a negative body image. You would not be reading this book if you did not want to improve something whether it's your weight, your confidence or your lifestyle and I will show you body image can affect your weight management.

In medicine and psychology, body image refers to a person's emotional attitude towards beliefs and perceptions about their own body. In other words, how a person feels about the way they look. When talking about feelings and perceptions, we're talking about something that is subjective rather than objective. For this reason, body image can be a complex issue. The important thing 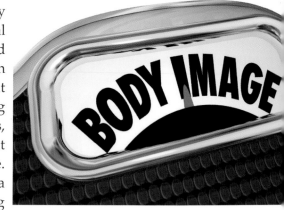 to remember about body image is that it's just an 'image' – it isn't necessarily based on reality and ideas about beauty and attractiveness change depending on the time period or culture you live in.

Look at masculine and feminine beauty throughout the ages. The Renaissance showed a more realistic, fuller-figured image of the female body than we are used to today. A fuller-figured body shape was still desirable through the 1800s when women wore tight corsets to emphasise their hips and waists. It wasn't until the beginning of the 1900s that a slender figure became more desirable. There has been a greater emphasis on a slimmer figure ever since, while the popularity of dieting and weight-loss programmes has exploded since the 1980s. The ideal female body began to move from reality in the 1990s with 'airbrushing' in advertising and magazines, which manipulates pictures of women to give them flawless complexions and unrealistic body proportions.

Masculinity too changed over time, though the desire for a powerful muscular body shape has always been as important as it is today. Though now, thankfully, it is accompanied by an emphasis on personal hygiene and grooming and sometimes even an interest in yoga and meditation.

In today's society, we are bombarded with images of the human body from magazines, smart phones, TV and billboards. It is estimated that people living in cities are exposed to over 5,000 advertising images every day and in 2012 it was estimated that companies spent £17.2 billion on advertising in the UK alone. So if we're surrounded by it, how can we get away from it? POSITIVE BODY IMAGE is the answer. Positive body image means overpowering the negative thoughts with positive ones. Those with a positive body image are comfortable and happy with their appearance and accept that their own appearance doesn't match up to the ideal put forward by the media or their community. If you get on the scales and find you have not lost anything it can be overwhelmingly disheartening. This is one reason why people slip back into old ways and give up on losing weight. Maintaining a positive body image will help you on your weight-loss adventure and help you change your lifestyle for the better. I know you will feel it after you have completed your journey.

There is no magic wand I can wave to turn negative body image thoughts into positive ones, but I can show and advise you on how to introduce you to a healthier way of looking at yourself and the body. The more you practice these new thought patterns the more they will encourage and motivate you, making you feel better about who you are. This will give you the inspiration and reinforce the belief that you have the confidence to lose weight. I will discuss weight-loss and the laws of attraction later as I believe this can also help.

POSITIVE BODY IMAGE TIPS

Focus on the aspects of your appearance you can change

List the things you like about you and keep re-reading it to give yourself praise and reassurance that you can achieve what you want to. Wear clothes that are comfortable and make you feel good. Purchase a new top or dress, which you aim to fit into, to give yourself motivation, and when you accomplish those goals your confidence and positivity will radiate and shine through.

Keep in mind what is interesting and unique about you

Make yourself a list of your qualities, ask friends and family what they think of you and why they chose to be your friend. Positive thinking helps massively as losing weight is not only a lifestyle change and physically demanding, it can be emotionally demanding too. Listening to compliments and seeing yourself as a unique person will overcome any negative thoughts and give you the morale boost you might need.

Recognise what is strong and healthy about your body

Write down your achievements. Write down what your best asset is. Recognising your strengths gives you the determination to overcome any weaknesses you have. Go for a walk. Walking is proven to be one of the best ways to express your thoughts. Everyone feels an energy spurt after working out in the gym; walking is a great way to clear your mind but also to be active and lose weight too!

Don't focus on what you cannot change

Be realistic. Your goal needs to be sensible, attainable and appropriate to your body. The media today is criticised for its continuous images and articles on weight-loss. Some argue that it causes men and women to have unrealistic expectations about their physical appearance and has directly contributed to the rise in eating disorders and dangerous dieting. Nowadays people are bombarded with airbrushed images of clinically underweight professional models that lead them to make unrealistic comparisons and set unnatural targets for personal change. Focus on your strong attributes and the list you have written about what you like about yourself. Focusing on unrealistic goals will only put doubt in your mind and lead to failure.

Give yourself compliments and eliminate self-criticism

Give yourself a compliment every day. Re-read your list about your positive qualities from family and friends. Eliminating self-criticism is hard, but look at the vision board you have made for yourself, look at it every day whether it is saved on your mobile phone, computer or pinned up on the wall. Write a spider diagram of what you love about yourself and look at it each day to fill yourself with the belief of the positive and beautiful person that you really are! Never mind that you are having a bad day, swap those negative thoughts for positive ones such as 'I may be struggling today but I had a good day yesterday and I've already lost three pounds this month.' Carry yourself with confidence.

Surround yourself with positive people

The attitudes of family and friends can be a major influence on someone's lifestyle. If we have friends who like to eat fast food and drink excessive amounts of alcohol, it can sometimes be hard not to do the same. Similarly, the habits of our families when we're growing up can influence our own habits in later life. If any of your family and friends are looking to lose weight or change habits in their lifestyle, then join up with them and do it together. This way you always have the support of each other. Join local community groups, maybe the gym, yoga classes, walking groups. There are so many places that offer activities for people like you. Just go somewhere you will feel supported and receive positive vibes as this will also increase your self-confidence and poise.

Use humour

Laughter is the best medicine. I know people who have used funny picture quotes to keep them motivated during their weight-loss journeys. Laughing is proven psychologically to put a person in a better mood. The weight-loss process will to be more enjoyable even if it is demanding at times if you keep a sense of humour. Keep laughing and it will not seem as challenging.

Hopefully these tips will help you on your journey and ultimately succeed with your lifestyle change. The next part of the chapter will discuss weight-loss myths and how the lifestyle choices you make affect weight management.

WEIGHT-LOSS MYTHS

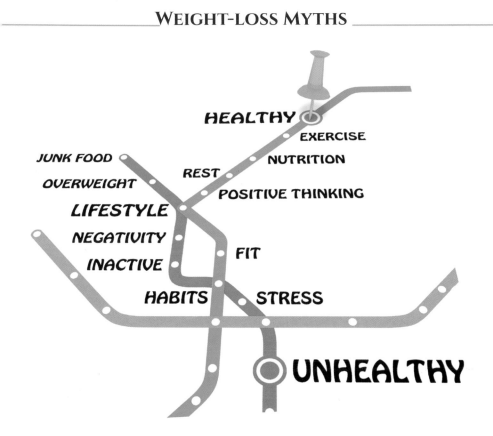

1. Starving yourself is the best way to lose weight

Starving yourself is not the best way to lose weight as it can cause harm and long-term weight gain. It is also too hard to maintain; because you're not eating the right nutrients, essential vitamins and minerals, your body will be so low on energy it will trigger cravings for high-fat sugary foods. When you eat these foods, consuming more calories than you actually need, you put on weight.

2. Radical exercise is the best way to lose weight

Adults between nineteen and sixty-four should get at least two and a half hours of physical activity such as fast walking or cycling weekly. Successful weight-loss includes making little changes that you can continue with over a long period of time. This means building regular exercise into your daily routine. For example, walking to work or the shops rather than driving. People who are overweight need to do this as they will struggle without implementing some type of physical activity. As discussed in a previous chapter you need to burn more calories than you eat or drink. Exercise and eating correctly is the only way to achieve this.

3. Slimming pills are a quick fix for losing weight

This could not be further from the truth and slimming pills, if not prescribed by a doctor, can be dangerous to your health. Slimming pills will be discussed further in the book as will the risks of taking them.

4. Healthy foods are more expensive

I hear this on a regular basis. People often assume healthy eating is expensive when in fact you pay more for fatty and sugary foods! Ask yourself: is it cheaper to purchase a banana or apple or a bar of chocolate? Organic fruit and vegetables can appear to be more expensive than purchasing a frozen meal, however frozen meals and processed foods are high in fat and salt, and vegetables and fruit can be purchased cheaply at markets.

5. Foods labelled 'low fat' or 'reduced fat' are always a healthy choice

This is a very clever marketing technique. How many times have you checked the labels of low-fat yogurts to find that while it may indeed be low in fat, it has a higher sugar content than the full-fat version? Not many chocolate manufacturers offer low-fat chocolate! If they did I am pretty sure we would all be snacking on it and not reading this book. Foods labelled 'low fat' have to meet specific legal criteria. Labels such as 'reduced fat' do not have to meet the same criteria and can be misinforming. This is why it is so important to read food labels and compare before you buy as this can often be misleading and confusing.

6. Margarine contains less fat than butter

Margarine and butter contain different types of fat. Margarine has less saturated fat than butter but is likely to contain hydrogenated fat that might be harmful to your health. A healthy diet should be low in both hydrogenated and saturated fats so, in terms of fat content, both are as bad as each other. If the oil in margarine has been hydrogenated, this has to be listed on the packaging, so again please check the labels to ensure you don't get confused.

7. Carbohydrates make you put on weight

Eaten in the right quantities, carbohydrates will not cause weight gain. Eat wholegrain and wholemeal carbohydrates such as brown rice and wholemeal bread, and don't fry starchy foods when trying to lose weight. You should eat carbs as they are an important part of our diet and low-carb diets do not sustain long-term results!

8. Cutting out all snacks can help you lose weight

Snacking isn't the problem when trying to lose weight: it's the type of snack. Instead of reaching for crisps and chocolate, go for a piece of fruit or some nuts, it will not do you any harm and will help you achieve your weight-loss goals more effectively than starving yourself.

9. You need to detox before you diet

Detoxing is not compulsory. Some people find it this helps them prepare for their weight-loss journey, while others believe that detoxing can be too challenging. It's personal preference, so do not believe that you have to do it. It is not part of the 'weight-loss law'. You make the rules and you do what suits you.

10. Skipping meals is a good way to lose weight

Skipping meals is not the best idea. To lose weight and keep it off, you have to reduce the number of calories you consume or increase the calories you burn through exercise. Skipping meals results in tiredness and poor nutrition. You will also be more likely to snack on high-fat and high-sugar foods, which could result in weight gain. If you are following a shake diet then you should still be receiving correct nutrition but, stay away from diets which give you shakes throughout the day and no food, this would just be foolish and your body will eventually crash and burn.

12. Drinking water can help with losing weight

Drinking enough water is essential to keep you fit and healthy. Water does not help you to lose weight, but it does keep you hydrated and could possibly help you snack less. You can confuse being thirsty for feeling hungry which can lead to snacking so before you eat, consider whether you might be thirsty.

Lifestyle choices

Are you always busy? Do you find it hard to eat healthily? This is quite common so don't think you're alone. I hear people say it almost every day. The truth is that if you are able to put a meal into a microwave for ten minutes you are almost certainly able to cook a healthy nutritious meal. How about eating out? Do you eat out regularly?

Let us take a look at ways in which we can change our thought processes when it comes to eating in restaurants. We are not saints and we should enjoy treats, but we spend more money and waste more calories by eating out. And it is hard to control your diet and eating habits if you cannot control the eating environment. Fast food is so readily available to us in today's society that eating out is the new normal. Years ago it was for special occasions, birthdays and treats, but today we think nothing of eating breakfast, lunch or dinner out. According to a survey from Allegra Strategies in 2013, 19 million adults eat out in the UK once a week compared to 2012 when this was 17 million a week and Allegra predict by 2018 the food industry is expected to be worth £90 billion. The convenience of takeaway outlets means people get into bad unhealthy habits, especially when they can order from websites offering a whole range of cuisines that can be delivered with a click of a button. How does this affect us? It becomes a habit. Maybe you start off with one takeaway night, say fish and chips on a Friday, then it because more regular because you've finished work late, don't fancy cooking or have possibly become addicted to bad food. I'm not saying don't eat out, we all need a treat, so I will introduce some tips and strategies to make it easier for us to choose healthier food. This particularly applies to those who eat out frequently. If you feel you are unable to cut back on eating out, then look at these tips and strategies to try and help you kick some of your old behaviours.

EATING OUT STRATEGIES

Selecting the restaurant

There are many choices, especially in cities, but you can still eat healthily while eating out. Be careful when choosing a place, for example a fish restaurant would be much healthier than an all-you-can-eat buffet and I am sure it would be much more appetizing. A place with a varied menu and plenty of choice would be better when eating out so that you are not limited in your options. Try thinking what you might like before you get to the restaurant, choosing on the spur of the moment often means picking the high fat option.

Before you leave for the restaurant

Take a look at the menu online before leaving home as it will give you an idea of the food the establishment serves. If the menu is full of fried foods then maybe go somewhere else as you know the battle will be lost the minute you walk through the door. Perhaps ask for a table away from the kitchen so you cannot see the other meals being brought as this might tempt you to change your mind about your choice. If you make a reservation, you won't be waiting around in the bar filling up on drinks and free snacks.

When you sit down

It is common for restaurants to offer free appetizers such as bread, bread sticks, butter, etc. The temptation is to eat them, so refuse them before you order or send them back if they arrive, otherwise they will fill you up before you get to the main meal. If you're feeling super strong-willed also give back the dessert menu so you won't be tempted to pick a pud. I don't mean you can't have three courses. If you only eat out once every blue moon then, of course, have three courses, but if you eat out more than once a week then you will only lose weight if you cut down on the size of your meal.

Game changers

When ordering, order first. I have been guilty of seeing my friends order before me and changing my mind because theirs sounds so much more delicious. Don't be afraid to ask for changes. You are the paying customer and it is your food even if you ask for a small portion! You can add veggies, load your plate with them! If you look for brightly coloured foods, you are on the right track. Unless, of course, it is a bright cake.

Starters – do not be fooled

You don't need to miss out on a starter but just consider the options. Garlic bread with cheese used to be my favourite until I discovered salad. Salad! I could eat it all I day long, I love it that much. Salads make a great starter but I usually ask for the dressing on the side. I am not a big lover of dressings and sauces but I know they are served with most foods and I am lucky I like plain food. Smoked salmon or seafood is another great healthy starter and so is soup but just make sure your soups are broth-based otherwise they could be loaded with calories.

Soups, salads and picky bits

We all love a good soup, however creamy soups are loaded with fat and calories, which is why I don't advise you to eat or cook them. Bean or pea soups are loaded with nutrients and fibre so to me this simple swap is worth it and they really are delicious. It's the same with salads; they add so many nutrients to a meal but the salad dressings do not! Tweaking the menu will not help you but also make you feel like you have the control to make informed decisions about foods.

Main courses – simple swaps

Avoid fried, pan-fried, creamed, buttered and breaded if you see these food choices on the menu. Instead go for steamed, grilled, boiled, poached, baked or stir-fried. These options are always better. Fatty meats to avoid are sausage, bacon, ribs and burgers. Opt instead for pork, chicken, turkey, fish and even steak if you ask for the fat to be cut off. Veggie options may appear healthy but always look at the sauce it is served with as this could be fattening – cheese sauce is popular with veggie options and often they are tossed in butter. If you are out for a special occasion, then do not feel you can't eat at all, but if you eat out regularly hopefully now you can see the effect it can have on you.

Side dishes

Steamed or boiled veggies are always the best option. I try to stick to veggies including sweet potato if this is available. Many people think coleslaw is a healthy option when in fact it's high in calories. Rice is fine if it is boiled and so are noodles! It comes down to making smart choices to load up on nutrients or you'll be defeating the object of losing weight.

Desserts – you can still eat them

Don't feel like you have to miss out on desserts. I love a good cake now and then, but if you eat them regularly then you are just asking the calories to pile onto you. I love frozen yogurts with fresh fruits which are a healthier choice than a big piece of chocolate cake loaded with cream. Be smart rather than greedy when ordering.

Helpful tips

Eating slowly is often a great way to feel fuller as you're giving your stomach time to make you feel fuller and digest your food. If you are chatting to friends, then you'll be focusing on the conversation and not on the food. Chewing gum also helps me feel full. You don't have to be a bore but if eating out is your hobby then some things need to change, so hopefully this section may have helped you change your thought processes around food.

CUISINE EATING AND WHAT TO AVOID

Chinese Restaurants

We all love a Chinese takeaway or meal but the problem in the UK is that Chinese meals are often deep-fried, not at all how the Chinese actually cook their meals. To stay motivated when eating in Chinese restaurants avoid deep-fried or battered dishes such as spring rolls, prawn toast and crispy seaweed. Ribs are also high in fat and salt and barbeque ribs are high in sugar. Watch out for fried dishes such as fried rice, sweet and sour dishes and the words 'crispy' or 'sizzling' as these are also likely to have been fried.

Foods to Order

Fish, fish and more fish on the condition it has been steamed. Dim sum has usually been steamed so I would recommend this and also stir-fried chicken and prawns with vegetables. All steamed or baked dishes are fine. Clear soups are great to have as a starter so you don't feel you are missing out and the best side dishes are boiled rice and noodles. Sauces are unavoidable so try to stick to low-sugar and low-salt sauces such as hot and sour. Having a sauce with your meal on one night is not going to break the calorie count, so maybe use this as a cheat night.

Indian restaurants

You can sample a range of recipes in Indian restaurants, however it can be easy to over-indulge. Indian main courses include curries with sauces. Some contain lots of cream, which we need to avoid so korma is off the list I am afraid. Again, avoid fried foods such as poppadums, bhajis and samosas. Sorry to be the bearer of bad news. The side dishes are the same as Chinese: avoid fried rice and pilau rice as they are fattening.

Foods to Order

The lovely curries with tomato bases. Indian restaurants often offer a range of vegetable dishes too, which is great as we love our veggies. Also I love the dishes cooked in a tandoor oven as they are fresh and tender, my favourites would be tandoori and tikka minus the sauces. Boiled rice would accompany my meal and for dessert stick to fresh fruit.

Thai food

Thai food is a lot healthier than Chinese food even though there are many similarities. The majority of Thai food, such as dim sum, poultry, fish and vegetables, is steamed. Try and avoid sauces made with coconut cream and deep-fried foods such as crispy noodles and spring rolls.

Foods to Order

Steamed dim sum, poultry, fish and vegetables. Thai restaurants serve steamed or boiled rice and any fish or meat that has been grilled. If you are unsure about sauces, don't be afraid to ask what is in them. They may just make you your own special sauce.

Italian food

Italian food is carbohydrate central but we don't need to avoid it as carbs are important. Nevertheless, there are particular things we could avoid. Try to avoid deep pan pizzas and those with stuffed crusts, also pizza toppings that contain processed meats, such as meatballs and pepperoni. Garlic bread is another one to avoid as it is usually smothered in cheese and fat. As are sauces that contain cream such as carbonara and lasagne as they are also heavy on the stomach.

Foods to Order

Pizzas which are thin and crispy and covered with healthy toppings such as fresh tomatoes, mushrooms, peppers, onions and chicken. You can create your own pizzas too, so design a healthy one. Vegetarian dishes are good as the majority are steamed or boiled. If you want a meal with sauce try to stick to tomato-based dishes and grilled chicken, pork or fish.

Mexican food

I love Mexican food and, believe it or not, many dishes are healthy for you. The avocado-based dip, guacamole, originates from Mexican food. However, I would steer clear of refried beans as well as tacos and tortillas as they are deep-fried.

Foods to Order

Soft tortillas are perfectly fine to eat so try some fajitas, which are cooked fresh and come in a variety of fillings. Enchiladas are also great too but just ask for less cheese. These are usually accompanied with salad or vegetables too which are great to fill up on. Vegetarian options are usually available in Mexican diners and contain beans and salsa which are tasty too.

Sushi restaurants

Sushi bars are the perfect place to eat out as the food is prepared healthily and is mostly fish. There is a variety of raw fish for you to taste – just avoid the sauces as they may be high in salt or sugar.

BARRIERS TO HEALTHY EATING

There are no barriers to healthy eating which cannot be overcome. Some of the barriers may be medical, involve work commitments or food allergies but there is always an alternative. There are so many people in this bracket who think they don't have choices but in reality they do! It is about discovering what options are available to you.

Cost

Many people believe it is more expensive to eat healthily and therefore choose to buy ready meals or convenience food. So you could purchase, for example, a packet of chocolate for a pound when you could get five bananas for the same price. If you visit a coffee shop then a bottle of water would be cheaper than a cup of coffee; in a restaurant a steak salad would be cheaper than steak and chips. It is simply a case of planning and finding alternatives. If you buy in bulk, prepare nutritious home-made meals in advance and freeze them it is actually cheaper to feed yourself and your family that way than it is by purchasing fatty ready meals. You cannot put a price on health and if you want to start a weight-loss journey this includes eating the right food groups. Keeping meals simple and cost effective is another way to do this. Many supermarkets today are in competition with one another to be the cheapest and this gives customers the advantage as they can shop around. Look for deals, discounts and coupons that give money off in stores. Look for the supermarket fruit and vegetables boxes which are relatively new and aimed at families. One will last you a week and I think it is an absolutely superb idea. If you worked out your weekly food budget and did your shop, then you would see how much cheaper fresh food is. This does not mean breaking the bank by going organic, just buying within your budget. Also add up the amount you spend on eating out and takeaways I am sure you will get a shock when you consider the ways your money could be better spent.

Information overload

There is so much confusing information on healthy eating, dieting and weight-loss. Everyday there are articles in newspapers and magazines, on the TV, internet and social media about healthy eating or the latest 'guaranteed results' celebrity diet. What you need to remember is that these new great celebrity diets are often without guidelines or medical information to help you. Then there are the contradictory articles in newspapers telling us one week that red wine, say, is bad for our health and then the next week that it is good. I can see how people get confused and how misleading information can have a negative effect on individuals' health.

Time Consuming

Many people say 'I don't have the time' and I don't condone this excuse at all. Make time! Not only do you say you want to lose weight but you need to consider your health. Not the next door neighbour's, or their cat's or your uncle's goldfish's, YOUR health and if you want to succeed at anything in life including weight-loss then YOU have to make time. You can prepare as I have mentioned throughout this book. You are able to make informed decisions as adults what you eat and what you do not. Don't let the time excuse in your way. Excuses don't help, so cancel the night you had planned with friends or the wine club and prep your meals for the week ahead. Prepping can take a maximum two hours of your day and the more experienced you become, the quicker you you'll be until it becomes a routine. Get the family involved by asking your partner or children to help: one person chops the vegetables and another cooks. Find a way, not an excuse!

Food intolerances

It can be difficult to achieve weight-loss if you have a food intolerance, but it is only as hard as you make it. There are so many foods you could use as an alternative to the foods or drinks you are allergic to or intolerant of. Learn how to look at food labels as discussed and discover what you can and cannot consume. Think nutrients – so if, for example, you are unable to eat bread or wheat, swap your loaf for wheat-free bread; if cow's milk is an issue switch to soy milk. Get to know your diet as part of your planning, research it, speak to your GP or even a dietician who will be able to help you they may even be able to give you a list of healthy foods which would help plan your weekly shopping list and meals. Always find a solution.

Changing habits

It is hard to change a habit. Studies have shown that it can take twelve weeks on average to form a new habit. Losing weight is not easy or we would all be thin matchstick people, but changing your thought processes makes changing your habits easier and this is how you overcome thought barriers. I have spoken already about changing our habits as I believe it is the most important method for losing weight and changing lifestyles. Habits that have taken years to build will not change in a day. Always ensure you can identify your triggers and have replacements ready to help you change.

Vegetarianism

If you are a vegetarian considering weight-loss, then bear in mind you need to make sure you are still getting the right amounts of nutrients for a healthy diet. Vegetarians are generally conscientious about what they eat and are often already eating healthily so as long as you are not going without, I am sure you can succeed on your weight-loss adventure.

Medication

Medication is a tough barrier to weight-loss, but my advice is to speak to your GP who may be able offer medication along with healthy eating plans tailored specifically to your needs. If you suffer with weight gain due to this my advice to you is do not give up. Doing something is better than doing nothing and every pound lost, or walk taken, is a step in the right direction.

Access to healthy food

If you have no transport, then it may be hard to access shops. However, you now have other options such as online shopping. If you have family or friends, then ask if they will take you along when they do their weekly shop. I am sure they would be more than happy to help and support you on your journey.

There are barriers and difficulties in life no matter what we do, but we always find ways to climb over the obstacles and get to the finish line and weight-loss is no different. If you make reasons not to do something, then you will never achieve or maintain your ideal weight.

MAKE AN EFFORT NOT AN EXCUSE!

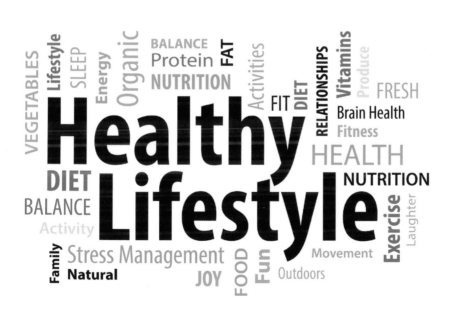

CHAPTER 5
WEIGHT-LOSS DIETS V LIFESTYLE CHANGE

'I am not dieting; I am changing my lifestyle'

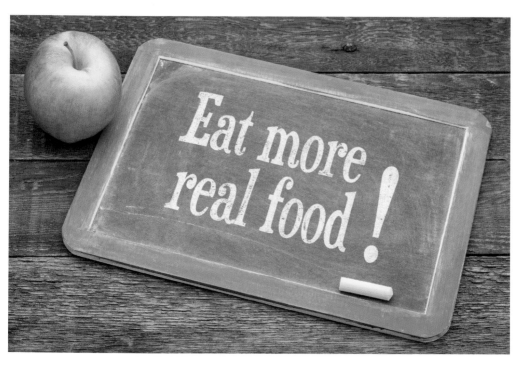

While healthy eating is becoming more popular around the world, especially in the UK and USA, where people are learning to give up unhealthy food for natural ingredients, there are always quick fix diets which offer solutions that are not sustainable in the long term. If you only wish to lose a few pounds they may work for you, but bear in mind you are likely to put the weight back on if they are too difficult to maintain.

The recommended calorie intake if you wish to lose weight is between 1,200-1,500 per day depending on your height and level of activity. Anything under that is considered unsustainable and could be dangerous in the long term, therefore I wouldn't suggest you follow a diet that recommends a daily intake of, say, 800 calories.

Nor would I recommend cutting out food groups altogether as it might mean you lose nutrients that will help you lose weight. The important aspect is changing your lifestyle and maintaining results through longterm healthy eating and regular exercise – consistency is key. In reality, any diet will work if it helps you take in a fewer calories, but will it work long term? This book is about changing your lifestyle so you no longer need these quick-fix diets.

Detoxing

The idea of detoxing is to rid of the toxins and chemicals from within the body for a period of time and is supposed to purify the liver, kidneys and bowel in particular. Detox diets can last anything from a day to a month and may involve fasting, restricting food consumption, cutting out certain food groups – such as dairy or wheat – and avoiding caffeine and alcohol. There are now even pills and bath products to help you detox. So does it work? The overwhelming evidence says no. Further it might make you dizzy and extra tired. Also any weight you lose won't be fat, it'll be water, stored carbs and muscle tissue. And if you are fasting or limiting your diet you won't be following a healthy eating plan, which is what we are aiming for.

As long as you are sensible, following a reputable short-term detox plan probably won't do you any harm and it might give you the kickstart you need, but once you stop you'll quickly put the weight back on unless you also change your lifestyle. It makes more sense to me to start straight in on the healthy eating and achieve sustainable weight-loss right from the start.

If you do a detox avoid alcohol, cigarettes, milk, sugar, coffee, saturated fats, wheat and dried fruits and go for foods such as fruit, vegetables, fish, meat, legumes, eggs, nuts, seeds, green tea and water – foods you'll be eating more of anyway once you start healthy eating. If you want to do a over-the-counter detox, make sure it is from a reputable supplier.

JUICING AND SMOOTHIE MAKING

Juicing has become extremely popular in the last few years. There are juicing cleanses, detoxes and smoothies which are available in shops or bars, and countless recipe books have been published showing you how to make them at home and alongside this there has been a huge increase in the sales of the latest juicing equipment and smoothie makers. But how good are juices for you? Well, like everything in life, there are pros and cons. There is not much medical research on the claims that juicing except that it might boost your immune system — however eating the whole fruit would also do that. Juicing companies have claimed that juicing can prevent illnesses such as cancer and dementia

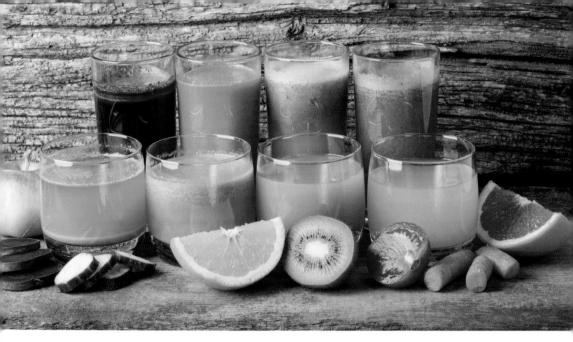

but as yet there is no medical evidence or studies to prove this. You may think that juicing is a great way to get fruit and vegetables into your diet and, if you struggle to eat these, can be a good short-term solution, however nutritional values may be reduced since juicing removes the nutrient-rich skin and pulp. Nutritionist Monica Reinagel of the Mayo Clinic which has conducted research says 'The antioxidants and other phytonutrients start to break down almost immediately once they are exposed to light and air.' Removing vital nutrients and fibre from your diet can reduce your body's ability to absorb fructose from fruit juice, which in turn can upset blood sugar levels and a lack of fibre leads to an unhealthy gut and even constipation. Since juices lack protein you could add almond milk, Greek yogurt or flaxseed.

Vegetable juices are better from a calorie point of view as they are lower and fruit smoothies can be high in sugar content as it takes more fruit to fill your glass than you would eat as a single serving.

Professor Barry Popkin from the Department of Nutrition in North Carolina University, and Dr George Bray, an American physician, have said that people are deceiving themselves . Professor Popkin said: 'Think of eating one orange or two and getting filled. Now think of drinking a smoothie with six oranges and two hours later it does not affect how much you eat. We feel full from drinking beverages like smoothies but it does not affect our overall food intake, whereas eating an orange does. So pulped-up smoothies do nothing good for us but do give us the same amount of sugar as four to six oranges or a large coke. It is deceiving.'

They say in recent published research that 'To the best of our knowledge every added amount of fructose – be it from fruit juice, sugar-sweetened beverages or any other beverage, or even from foods with high sugar content – adds equally to our health concerns linked with this food component.' Research from the British

Medical Association, published in 2016, also found that nurses who ate whole fruit in particular blueberries, grapes and apples were less likely to get type 2 diabetes, but those who drank fruit juice were at increased risk. The research also discovered that while the consumption of sugary drinks had fallen by 9 per cent over the last ten years, obesity had risen by 15 per cent. It seems there is so much disagreement around diets and healthy eating, so what is the ideal way to juice?

My personal opinion is that if you don't consume any fruit and vegetables within your diet then this is a great way of sneaking them back in and it helps retrain your taste buds to enjoy fruits and veggies again. Nutritionist Jennifer Barr from Wilmington, Delaware suggests that you should mix the colours of your fruit and vegetables in your juices so that you are getting a good mix of different vitamins and minerals. She also suggests that to avoid missing out on your fibre intake you should add the pulp back into the juice or use it when cooking dishes such as soup or rice. Smoothies and juices are fun to make and you can be creative with them, they are popular with children as the whole family can get involved to become healthier. Not only can they be beneficial to health in moderation, they can also be great for improving hair, skin and nails due to the antioxidants and phytonutrients contained within the fruits.

If you are thinking of making the occasional juice or smoothie use a good blender which retains the fibre and protein instead of an expensive juicer. My belief is that if you have juices in moderation as with any other food or drink then you are doing no harm. I have given you a few of my favourites which I enjoy making and which taste delicious too.

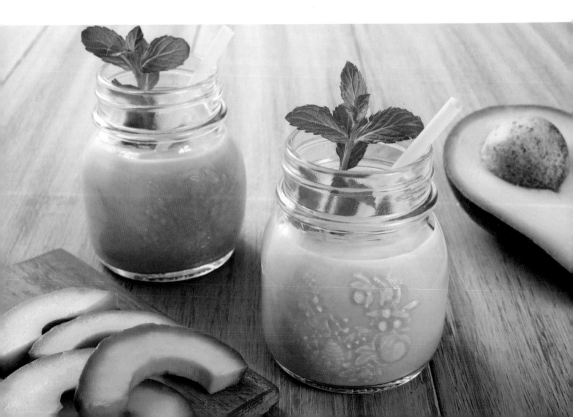

Smoothie recipes for you and for the whole family

Avocado Delight

I banana
Handful of kale
I kiwi fruit
1/2 avocado
400ml milk
Itbsp honey

Then blend together until contents are smooth and stir for a super delicious taste.

Banana and Berry Delight

1/2 cup vanilla yogurt
3/4 cup apple juice
I banana
3/4 cup frozen blueberries
1 1/2 cups frozen strawberries

Chop up the banana into chunks. Stick in a blender for sixty seconds until ingredients are smooth and creamy.

All you can eat fruit smoothie

1/4 cup of strawberries
1/4 cup of blueberries
1/2 apple chopped up
1/4 cup of mango
I banana
400 ml cow's milk or rice milk if lactose intolerant
I tablespoon of seeds: pumpkin, flax, goji berries

Chop up the fruit and add to a blender to create a great nutritious smoothie.

Peach melba

75g / ¾ cup frozen raspberries
240ml / I cup almond milk
Itsp vanilla extract
Itbsp lemon juice
I peach, peeled and chopped
240ml / I cup orange juice

Chop up the peach and add together all the ingredients for a lovely refreshing peach tasting smoothie!

Spinach galore

 1 tbsp coconut oil
 2 cups organic spinach
 1 cup organic frozen strawberries
 1 small frozen banana
 1 tbsp organic peanut butter
 1 cup filtered water

Mix together in a blender until smooth

Mango madness

 8 pieces or 3/4 frozen mango about ¾ cup
 1/2 cup coconut milk

Add into a blender. Blend until smooth. Then add one tablespoon chia seeds and pulse to create a thicker smoothie

---

To make a smoothie you can use any ingredients to create a super delicious taste! To make it more fun, you could hold a smoothie-making night in your house and ask family and friends over. Think about the ingredients you are putting in and how they will benefit you. I have listed ten top ingredients which I think are perfect, along with the reasons they are so good for us!

Leafy greens – spinach, kale, etc

These lower our cholesterol and are high in vitamin and minerals which help give us energy and fuel our body. Their high levels of calcium help keep our bones healthy. They are also good for our eye sight and in reducing the risk of type 2 diabetes. I think smoothies are a superb way to sneak leafy greens into our five a day.

Berries

The antioxidant boom. Berries are full of antioxidants, which help with good health and are amazing for our skin. Raspberries, blueberries, blackberries and strawberries: you name any berry and it has a purpose. Not only do they taste delicious but they are low in sugar and low in calories since they are mostly water based.

Avocado

Green or black, this fruit is great for energy boosts and it contains good mono-saturated fat too. Avocado is discussed later in the superfoods section.

Bananas

A tropical fruit which is delicious and a great healthy snack. High in potassium and fibre with high sugar levels means they are a great snack when you need an energy boost. Try a banana smoothie if you miss breakfast or even as a snack in the afternoon.

Almond milk

Great alternative to cow's milk. With the option of sweetened and unsweetened, you can choose the taste of your smoothie, plus it's great for those who are lactose intolerant. Almonds are also a healthy food full of vitamins, minerals as well as healthy fats and fibre.

Flax seeds or hemp seed

These both deliver a delicious nutty flavour, fibre and a healthy serving of essential fatty acids. Ensure that you grind the seeds too so you are getting the full nutrients from each serving. Adding these to smoothies and breakfast cereals will quickly become a habit that you won't even need to think about.

Yogurt

Natural or organic live yogurt without high-fructose corn syrup would be the best. It is a great alternative to milk.

Raw honey

An amazing natural sweetener which is underestimated. If you added this to a smoothie it would give you sweet-tooth dieters the perfect taste you need.

Apples

An apple a day keeps the doctor away. I love apples. Did you know there are numerous varieties of apples all with different flavours? It is also a low-glycaemic fruit that is a great source of fibre.

Coconut water

Great alternative to milk, an incredible source of electrolytes and a great way to dilute the consistency of your smoothie. It is also low in calories, cholesterol free and super hydrating.

Also don't forget ice cubes! Nothing tastes better or more refreshing than a cold smoothie! And ice cubes are calorie-free!

MEAL REPLACEMENT PLANS

Also known as shake diets, these arrived on the scene over fifty years ago but in the last few years there has been a dramatic increase in new brands and manufacturers. Shake diets are usually meal replacements often for breakfast or lunch or both, sometimes also the evening meal, where the shake itself contains the nutrients, proteins and carbohydrates. Most people do not need to follow this kind of diet, since a balanced healthy eating plan will be enough to help them lose weight. However, if you do need to, you should follow the instructions carefully and follow it for no longer than twelve continuous weeks. If you are using it intermittently alongside healthy nutritious meals then you can go for longer. Critics say that meal replacements are a quick fix and dieters will put any weight lost straight back on, however, they could be a good way for people to help regain control over overeating and give them the push to start pursuing a healthy lifestyle. Obviously you need to keep this healthy lifestyle up when you finish your shake diet or it will defeat the object of the exercise. If you struggle to get started with any diet at all then a shake diet or a smoothie could help you. You should not become reliant on these diets as you still need healthy sources of food and an active lifestyle. Steven Heymsfield and MD of St Luke's Roosevelt Hospital found that using diet shakes to replace one to two meals a day can assist in losing 7 to 8 per cent of body weight in one year. It is down to you to research the shakes you want to consume, just remember brands of shake vary in their balance of carbohydrates, fats, proteins and vitamins and minerals which is why you should check with a professional if unsure.

Supplements

The American Food and Drug Administration (FDA) defines a supplement as:
    'A product intended for ingestion that contains a "dietary ingredient" intended to add further nutritional value to (supplement) the diet. Dietary ingredients may be one or a combination of the following substances: a vitamin, mineral, herb or other botanical, amino acid, dietary substance, a concentrate, metabolite, constituent or extract.'
    If you search the web for supplements thousands of results appear including those for weight-loss, vitamins and minerals, protein, natural and organic, body building, fish oils and those which claim to prevent or treat common colds, so which to take, if any? In the West most of us get enough nutrition through our diet and so we don't need to take supplements. So if they are unnecessary why do people take them? Possibly because they don't like to miss out on anything they believe might give them better health, prevent ageing or ease illness. Others believe modern farming methods and the use of chemicals as fertilisers prevent foods from containing the full amount of vitamin and minerals. They think a

safe and effective supplement may help with this. Others still might have poor absorption of vitamins and minerals because of illness or medication – if this is you, you should talk to your doctor first. The average healthy person with a healthy balanced diet doesn't need to take supplements. The Medicines and Healthcare Regulatory Agency is responsible for ensuring that medicines are safe, and mostly they are, but it is highly difficult to ensure the compliance of any unscrupulous online retailers. So if you wish to take supplements the best option is to go to a reputable health outlet either on the high street or online as they can only sell products which have been tested. If in doubt always check the label and speak to an assistant before purchasing.

As well as remembering the NHS's advice it is worth noting that of the thousands of claims submitted to the European Food Safety Authority around 80 per cent of supplement health claims are declined. I will now cover some of the basic supplements which people generally consume and how they are rated by professions.

Vitamins and minerals

Use food labelling to assess which vitamins are best for you. Firstly, look for labels which say '100 per cent natural'. The Organic Consumer's Association recommends anything which declares itself 100 per cent plant based or 100 per cent animal based on the product label, otherwise you could be buying man-made products. If the label does not show the list of natural food sources then this means the product is synthetic. Food sources that you should look for are yeast, vegetables and fish. Next look for specific salt forms. The main ones to look out for are acetate, gluconate, nitrate and chloride. If you are unsure, then speak to your GP or a nutritionist who can help you make the decision. Bear in mind that vitamins are not always harmless when taken in large quantities. And overdosing on them can cause side effects including abdominal pain, weight-loss, vomiting, headaches and blurred vision. Vitamin C is a good example – it is the UK's most popular single vitamin and the annual sales total £36 million. The EU recommends that the daily intake should only be 80mg and the dangers of taking vitamin C supplements can be the rise of blood sugar levels, which is especially dangerous for those with diabetes. According to the NHS you should also avoid effervescent tablets as they can contain 1g of salt, which is not ideal if you're trying to cut back on your salt intake.

There are no super pills which will beat eating the real whole foods, nevertheless, I do believe that vitamin supplements can help for a short period and particularly with those who are struggling with vitamin deficiencies or those who are still working out how to balance their diets, but I cannot stress enough how important it is to check with a health professional especially if you have an existing medical condition or are pregnant.

Fish oil supplements

The omega fats and fatty acids these supplements provide, and which we need for our health, can only be obtained by eating fish oils as they are not made by the body. These supplements are not suitable for everyone as they can react with certain medications and be dangerous for pregnant women. I would advise they are suitable for those who can't get omega fats and fatty acids into their diet in other ways such as by eating a nice piece of salmon. There is no medical evidence that taking fish oil supplements boosts brain power.

Slimming pills

I would avoid these at all costs. They supposedly curb your cravings for food, make you feel full before you have eaten too much, speed up your metabolism, slow down your body's fat production or keep your body from absorbing fat! This, I would suggest, is all too good to be true – if it wasn't surely every GP would be prescribing them for the rising obesity problem. The issue is that many of these pills are available through the internet and are often unregulated, so it is difficult to know if they are safe. Unscrupulous manufacturers certainly won't tell you the potential dangers of using them such as increased heart rate, high blood pressure, agitation, vomiting, diarrhoea, insomnia, kidney problems, liver damage, rectal bleeding, heart attacks and strokes. In America, the FDA have found pills containing medications to help with seizures, blood pressure medication and prescription-only anti-depressants such as fluoxetine. They also found that pills which were claiming to be '100 per cent natural' contained toxic ingredients and a banned substance called sibutramine. These diet products are not recommended for those who are normal weight or underweight and can be extremely dangerous for people with eating disorders. Beware when you see weight-loss products being advertised and avoid anything promising a quick fix; or that makes claims which seem to good to be true; those are written in a language you can't read or therefore understand, or anything marketed through spam. Because these products are so easily obtained on the internet, it is extremely difficult for medical and health care agencies to control their sale and my advice is that it is not worth the hassle unless they are being prescribed by a doctor or on the advice of a health care professional.

The gluten-free diet

Everyone, including many celebrities, has gone crazy over gluten-free diets. NPD, a marketing research company in America, has said 29 per cent of Americans (that's 70 million people) tried to cut gluten from their diet in 2014, and it was just as popular in the UK – a report from Mintel showed that sales from the UK of gluten-free products reached £184 million in the same year, up by 15 percent from 2013. So what is gluten? Gluten is a protein found in wheat, barley and rye, which can all cause sensitivity in the bowel and digestive system and also bloating of the stomach. It is also linked to coeliac disease. People who have coeliac disease follow a gluten-free diet and how happy they must be now this diet has risen in popularity. Years ago, gluten-free foods used to be on prescription, now supermarkets have special sections offering a much wider selection. People who follow a gluten-free diet are able to eat most foods such as meat, fish, fruit, vegetables and potatoes. Those they cannot eat, or are advised to steer clear of, are beer, breads, cakes, cereals, gravy, pies, processed meats, pastas, sauces including salad dressings, soups and sweets. So now can you see why it is becoming so popular: the foods listed above are exactly what people want to cut out on a regular diet which is low in carbohydrate and high in protein. But is all gluten-free produce good for us? Gluten-free foods replace those foods gluten intolerant people are unable to consume, so what are manufacturers replacing it with? Research has shown that substitute foods may be free of gluten, but they are often higher in sugar and fat, which cause weight gain. Also by eating a gluten-free diet you are reducing your intake of fibre from wholegrains and carbohydrates. Unless you are suffering from conditions such as celiac disease or dermatitis herpetiformis, this won't lead to weight-loss and therefore it is probably not the diet for you. There have been reports of individuals stating that they have increased energy from this diet, but there are no studies to support this and this could simply be that they receiving the energy from swapping fruit and vegetables for high-calorie processed food. Another point to consider is that gluten-free food is a lot more expensive and takes a lot more time and dedication. Lack of time and dedication are usually why people fail at diets in the first place so why would someone stick to this if they can't to stick to a healthy, balanced diet? With this in mind I believe that removing gluten from your diet has no direct effect at all and I would only recommend this diet to those who really need it. Trend diets often appear an easier option than sticking to regular, nutritious meals; this is not usually the case.

Home remedies

We all know old wives' tales that supposedly help us get rid of the common cold, unblock noses and, of course, help us lose weight. I will discuss some of the favourite remedies I have come across in the last few years and why they may work. Again there is no long-term medical evidence to support them but they may just help you on your weight-loss journey. Dieting and weight-loss are all learning curves and, since they aren't high in calories or sugar, they might just be a great alternative your usual drinks.

Lemon juice – great for detox and improving digestion. Can aid with detoxing, and while there's no evidence to show that this can help with weight-loss, this drink would be ideal before starting a diet, just so you can detox your whole body and prepare for the lovely change.

Cinnamon tea – blood sugar plays an important part in weight-loss as it influences how hungry you are and how energetic you are feeling. I would encourage any tea lovers to swap their cup of cha to a cup of this.

Alternative therapies

Many people use alternative therapies to help lose weight, which work for some and not for others. Individuals may choose to use these alongside their diets or lifestyle changes to assist them. So what are these therapies you may be asking.

The US National Centre for Complementary and Integrative Health (NCCIH) uses this distinction:

When a non-mainstream practice is used together with conventional medicine, it's considered 'complementary'.

When a non-mainstream practice is used instead of conventional medicine, it's considered 'alternative'.

Alternative therapies all share the belief that the body is able to heal itself. This could be through a variety of remedies such as aromatherapy, acupuncture or reiki. I will discuss a few alternative therapies and what they are and their approaches to helping with weight-loss.

Firstly, acupuncture. Acupuncture is a Chinese healing approach based on positive and negative energies circulating round the human body. The theory is that if the flow of these energies is blocked, imbalances occur which will then manifest as health problems such as obesity. Acupuncture is intended to restore this balance through the insertion of thin needles into the skin at pre-determined points. This then stimulates the tissues within the body ease the blockages and restores the energy flow. This treatment can also be used for pain relief, headaches and even addiction. How it may be able to help with weigh loss is by reducing your hunger and cravings.

Next is acupressure it is essentially acupuncture without the needles, where the strategic points are stimulated through finger pressure and it has the same effect.

Thirdly, hypnosis. In this therapy trained clinical hypnotists use a variety of techniques such as guided visualisation to improve an individual's self-image and hypnotic proposals to make their life healthier. It also aims to change thought patterns to encourage patients to follow a healthy and nutritious diet plan, as well as creating a tranquil frame of mind. This is good for those who use food when stressed, anxious or depressed and it is beneficial for the mind and body as it relaxes a person and removes bad energy. I have a friend who used hypnotherapy after trying various diets and who admitted she had no self-control or willpower regarding food – everything around her was temptation. After three sessions with a hypnotherapist looking at her habits around and perceptions of food and what she felt she would like to remove from her diet, she changed her eating patterns and chose to exercise. When she got cravings she took her mind off them by doing something she she enjoyed and this helped her not only lose weight, but to continue on her healthy journey learning to cooking healthy meals and increasing her physical activity levels daily.

Like other alternative therapies, reiki uses the same theory of removing negative energy from the body and balancing the energy flow, so practitioners who are qualified in reiki use their positive energy to stimulate natural healing in the body. This does not involve any significant physical contact, just light touching or hands hovering over you projecting energy. There are energy centres throughout your body called chakras, which are each represented by a different colour and connect to your body's overall being. A chakra may be blocked due to illness or injury, which then causes additional problems so practitioners who use reiki must stimulate self-healing. I use this treatment when I am stressed as it relaxes me and restores my sleep pattern. It has also helped my manage a back condition – it does not cure it, but helps me think of other ways I can focus on it if I am ever in pain. I am not going to suggest this will definitely work for you as each individual is different, however there are no bad side effects from this treatment, only good ones and as you are not consuming food, supplements or any form of medication there is no danger of bad physical side effects such as diarrhoea or vomiting.

There are seven main chakras: the three which affect your weight are the spleen, solar plexus and throat. If one of these is out of alignment, there's an imbalance such as depression, diabetes, lack of confidence or digestive problems, which might lead to weight gain. Reiki can aid weight-loss by making you more aware of your body. When people feel stressed or anxious or have low confidence they tend to crave food and overeat. This spiritual treatment can help lift your mood and stabilise your appetite, making you aware of the nutritional needs of your body. It can often help you see things differently by making you feel better about yourself, bringing out the positive energy which gives you the boost to want to lose weight. It can also prevent a build-up of stress hormones such as cortisol that is known to affect weight. If you choose to opt for reiki as an alternative therapy, always speak to a qualified practitioner and explain which imbalance you would like to overcome.

None of these therapies will help you directly in losing weight but they may increase your sense of well-being and encourage you on your journey. And they are extremely enjoyable.

Weight-loss wraps

Have you ever seen a local beauty salon or individual advertising a wrap that can help take inches off your body? They are becoming more and more popular. Studies have found they will work for a short period of time but they are pricey and results are not maintained. They're not really about weight-loss, but if you are looking to lose inches before a big event these would work, but don't be surprised if the lost inches reappear afterwards. Sandra Fryhofer, MD at the American College of Physicians says, 'any loss of inches is going to be temporary, wraps cannot take the place of a healthy diet and exercise.' So they may make you feel thinner for a short amount of time and they are very pampering, but always speak to a consultant or therapist before trying one and ask to see evidence of results.

The Mediterranean diet

This is not a fad diet but rather a healthy lifestyle change and incorporates foods are beneficial to your weight-loss journey. It has been the traditional of countries bordering the Mediterranean Sea such as Italy, France, Spain, Turkey and even Morocco for centuries and incorporates the basics of healthy eating as it advocates consuming mainly fruits and vegetables, wholegrains, legumes and nuts. The grains that you consume as part of this diet have very few unhealthy trans fats and, although bread is an important part of the diet, it is eaten plain without butter. Red meat should be limited to only a few times a month and fish and poultry should be consumed twice a week. Butter and margarine is replaced

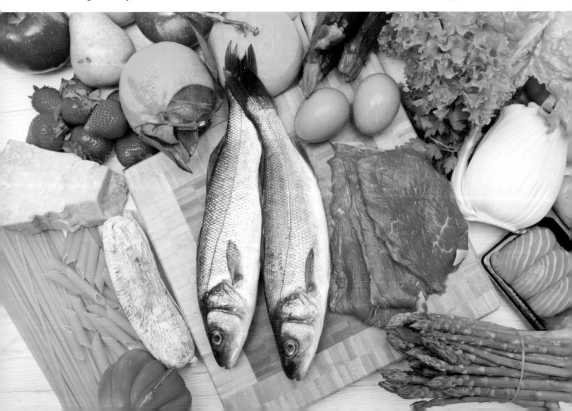

by olive oil and instead of salt you should use herbs and spices to flavour your foods. Drinking red wine is also included in this diet recommendation, however this is optional. Physical exercise is important too, which is great as this shows this is not a quick fix but really a lifestyle change. One big factor of this diet, in fact one of its key components, which I think is different to other diets, is it is about enjoying meals with family and friends. A big part of society's problem today regarding food is that our busy social lives and work schedules prevent us eating together as a family. Research has shown that the traditional Mediterranean diet reduces the risk of heart disease and, in an analysis of more than 1.5 million healthy adults, it established that it also reduced risk of cancer and Alzheimer's. The NHS explains that this diet is similar to that set out by the government in the Eatwell Plate. In 2003, a study published in the New England Journal of Medicine and conducted in Spanish universities showed that of the 7,447 people who took part and followed the Mediterranean diet, 30 per cent had a reduced risk of suffering a heart attack or stroke.

So what are the pros and cons. I will be honest: I cannot find many cons. So many countries including the USA and UK agree this diet is so great that they have built their own recommendations around it. Firstly, there is no calorie counting; this diet is literally a way of life. Freshly-cooked food is the best way to a healthy diet, however it is much easier for people to purchase readymade meals and processed food rather than vist the local market or buy fresh from a supermarket or deli.

In Italy, a village called Campodimele is dubbed 'the village of eternal youth' by scientists as the life expectancy here averages ninety-five years. They cultivate all their own foods and do not have any packaged foods. They pickle their own vegetables and use seasonal ingredients to cook their fresh meals, which they flavour with herbs and spices instead of salt. This gives massive health benefits since these have been shown to be health-boosting foods. Rosemary and coriander are two of these seasonings which contain disease-fighting antioxidants and other nutrients. Whoever would have thought we would have found a diet where fat is allowed? Well this is it. However, this fat is good fat such as olive oil rather margarine or butter. As well as using olive oil on bread they use it for salad dressing and make their own instead of buying, rather than pre-prepared dressings which are full of salt. This diet is extremely varied and below you will find some recipes I made when researching it. The variety is probably one reason why people don't get bored of cooking this type of food. You could also say it is expensive, but more often than not it is cheaper to buy fruit than sugary snacks and the health benefits are invaluable. So although this diet is not specifically designed for weight-loss, it has been shown that you will not be hungry as quickly if you follow it, since you will digest more slowly and the fibre it contains will make you feel less hungry. Evidence from France may be able to back this up as the French have lower rates of heart disease and cholesterol than other nations even though they love wine and cheese. They also take much longer to eat their meals than others in the EU: they have over an hour to sit and enjoy their food slowly rather than being on the go all of the time. Unfortunately the rest of us cannot always choose our meal breaks and have to make do with what we are given.

Although alcohol in moderation has been associated with reduced risk of heart disease, wine could be seen as possibly the biggest disadvantage to this diet due to the risks associated with it. However, it is optional and you can always swap it for water.

So we can learn many valuable lessons from this delicious diet – let us take a look at some dishes.

MEDITERRANEAN DISHES

Paprika cauliflower

Unique and different, this dish is great served alongside grilled fish or meat.

Ingredients

    1 cauliflower, cut into small florets
    3tbsp olive oil
    2tbsp paprika
    1/2tsp ground black pepper
    1 small red onion, diced (1 cup)
    1 clove garlic, minced (1tsp)
    1/2 cup low-sodium vegetable broth
    2tbsp lemon juice

Preparation

1. **Steam cauliflower until tender and soft** – approximately nine minutes in a non-stick pan, heat the oil, paprika and pepper on medium-low heat for two minutes while stirring constantly. Add in the onion and garlic, and sauté for two minutes more. Stir in the broth and cauliflower, and simmer for three minutes. Remove from heat, and stir in the lemon juice.

Olive, eggs and tuna salad

Seems bland but believe me it is delicious and quick to prepare. It is simple, effective and ensures you get your protein and omega fats in one super meal.

Ingredients

  1 small red onion, peeled and thinly sliced
  White or rice wine vinegar, as needed
  1 yellow pepper, seeded and chopped
  8 radishes
  12 olives, green and black, mixed
  2 hardboiled eggs cut into quarters
  1 small tin of tuna, drained
  1 tbsp capers

For the dressing
  1 tsp lemon zest
  1 tbsp fresh lemon juice
  4 tbsp olive oil
  Freshly ground black pepper

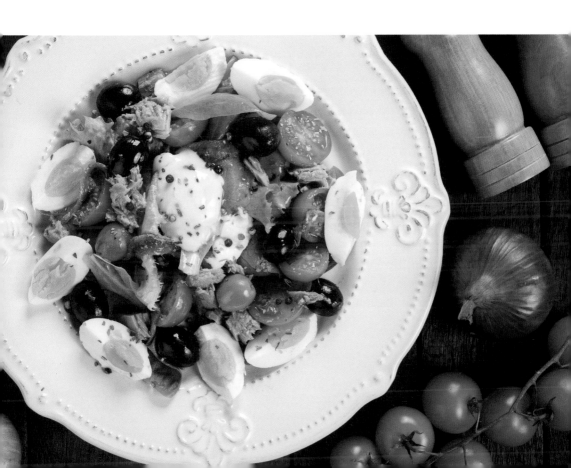

■ *Preparation*

1. Create the dressing by mixing the lemon zest, juice, oil and some freshly ground pepper within a bowl. Whisk until smooth and well blended.
2. To make the salad, toss together onion slices in a few tablespoons vinegar and set aside. On a large plate, position the peppers, radishes and place the olives around the edge. Arrange the eggs attractively in clusters of twos or threes, and mound the tuna in the middle. Sprinkle the capers over the tuna. Drain the onions and toss them over the salad. Add your dressing and some black pepper to season. You can always add additional items such as lettuce and tomatoes to make it more colourful.

Greek skewers

Great as a lunch or snack, maybe even turn this dish into a main meal by adding some rice and salad.

*Ingredients*_____

2tbsp extra virgin olive oil
1/2tsp dried oreganoz
2oz. feta, cubed
1 lemon, cut into 6 wedges
2 slices of Italian bread, cut into 16 1-inch cubes
16 cherry tomatoes
1/2 red onion, cut into one inch cubes
Romaine lettuce
1 cucumber, sliced
12 assorted pitted olives

■ *Preparation*

1. Soak eight bamboo skewers in water for around thirty minutes.
2. Mix the feta, oil and oregano together in a bowl. Drizzle two lemon wedges over the top to flavour.
3. Put the tomatoes and onion onto skewers. Glaze with olive oil spray and grill, turning carefully until golden brown – around four minutes.
4. Place the lettuce on four plates and put two skewers on top of each. Divide the cucumber, olives and feta mixture among plates and serve with the remainder of the lemon wedges.

Greek-style marinated chicken

Delicious and also refreshing. Perfect for a summer barbecue too.

Ingredients

120ml extra virgin olive oil
3 cloves of garlic
1tbsp rosemary
1tbsp thyme
1tbsp oregano
2 lemons
4 medium chicken fillets

■ *Preparation*

1. Squeeze the lemons. Cut the chicken into small pieces. Chop the fresh herbs. Crush the garlic.
2. In a glass dish, mix the olive oil, garlic, rosemary, thyme, oregano and lemon juice. Place the chicken pieces in the mixture, cover and marinate in the refrigerator eight hours or overnight.
3. Heat grill to a medium heat.
4. Lightly oil the grill with olive oil. Place the chicken on the grill and discard the marinade. Cook chicken pieces for fifteen minutes, turning halfway through until juices run clear, then serve with a side dish of your choice.

So after looking at the Mediterranean diet, let us now look at other diets from around the world and how their tried and tested diets may help us to a healthy nutritious, non-fattening diet. This is a really interesting section as there are so many health properties to these diets that we do not think about.

FOODS AROUND THE WORLD

Just as we have incorporated the Mediterranean diet into our cuisine, we can also bring in foods from other countries since we have access to a wide variety of multi-cultural foods and ingredients supermarkets and health shops.

Diets, as mentioned before, can become boring if we are eating the same foods and not introducing new ways to make them fun. We eat foods from other cultures in restaurants, takeaways in our homes when we make curries and paellas and when we are abroad we eat the local cuisine as part of the pleasure of being on holiday. So why not bring them into our weight-loss plan? After all, what foods do we have which inspire other countries? Pie and mash, fish and chips, toad-in-the-hole, Cornish pasties, full English breakfasts – not exactly the healthiest of options. The healthy meals we have are stews and a Sunday roast dinner but we also have a sweet tooth and we have a variety of English desserts such as spotted Dick and Victoria sponge. On the whole we don't go abroad and see our recipes being served in restaurants – not unless you are in an area popular with British tourists. Weight-loss is not just about calories, it is about educating ourselves on the foods we should be eating and introducing new ingredients so we don't become bored, which is the downfall of many people who start diets.

So let us look into countries around the world for tips, advice and inspiration that we could combine into our lifestyles. In some cases we are already doing this without even knowing, so let us become more knowledgeable and investigate other new foods.

You would think that countries such as the UK, USA, Australia would have great diets due to the knowledge we have about healthy eating and because we have access to a variety of fresh, nutritious ingredients. But often we are so busy in life that it is so much more convenient to buy ready meals and processed foods and shockingly our hospitals still see admissions from lack of nutrition as well as eating disorders, diabetes, strokes and cardiovascular diseases, even though the risk of all these diseases can be dramatically reduced through healthy eating. Here are some healthy recipes from around the world we could borrow.

Kimchi

South Korea's national dish is a side dish of fermented vegetables. Serve in a pancake or alongside grilled meat or fish

Ingredients

    1 cup medium cabbage, chopped
    1 cup carrots, thinly sliced
    1 cup cauliflower, separated into small pieces
    2tbsp salt
    2 green onions, thinly sliced
    3 cloves garlic, thinly chopped, or 1tsp garlic powder
    1tsp crushed red pepper
    1tsp fresh ginger, finely grated, or 1/2tsp ground ginger

■ *Preparation*

1. Combine the cabbage, carrots and cauliflower and salt in strainer.
2. Toss together lightly and leave in the sink for about an hour to drain.
3. Rinse with cold water, drain well and place in a medium-sized bowl.
4. Add the onions, garlic, red pepper and ginger and mix thoroughly.
5. Cover and keep in the fridge for at least two days, stirring occasionally.
6. Allow to sit for a further two days to ferment. If you want it spicier then let it sit for longer.

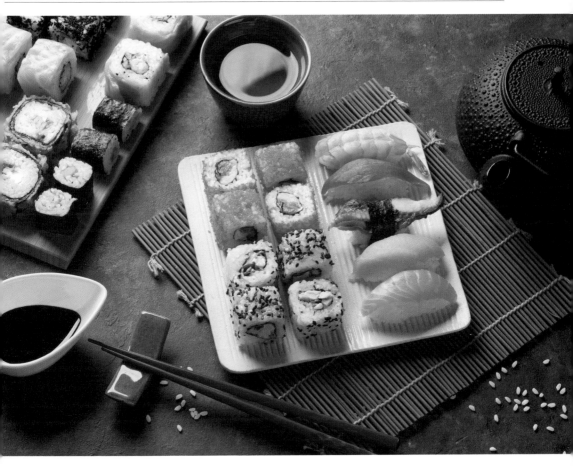

Tuna sushi roll

The Japanese have one of the best diets in the world. They eat 150 pounds of fish a year, mostly as either sushi or sashimi.

Ingredients

Tuna fillet cut into strips
Strips of carrot and cucumber
Sushi RicE
Nori (dry seaweed sheets)
Wasabi

Preparation

1. Place a sheet of nori (dry seaweed), shiny side down, on a makisu (bamboo mat).
2. Wet your right hand in the bowl of vinegar water, and use it to scoop up a ball of rice.
3. Spread the rice out in an even layer on one side of the nori.

4. Down the centre of the rice sprinkle a line of wasabi.
5. Arrange the strips of vegetables and tuna strips over the line of the wasabi.
6. Using the mat to support the seaweed sheets, lift one end of the mat to gently roll the seaweed sheets over the rice and other ingredients.
7. Use gentle pressure to compact the rice and other ingredients so that they are held firmly together.
8. Continue rolling until a long cylinder shape is formed, completely enclosed in the seaweed sheets.
9. Carefully slice through the seaweed sheets and other ingredients to make little bites of sushi.

Dal

Indian food incorporates a lot of vegetables and can be healthy if you steer clear of creamy sauces and deep-fried dishes. If you are eating out go for tandoori dishes and plain – not pilau – rice and dal. Dal is easy to make at home and it freezes well. This recipe makes ten to twelve portions.

Ingredients:

6 large onions
10 cloves of garlic
About a 2 inch piece of ginger
5 green chilis
10 big handfuls of green lentils (soaked over night or at least thirty mins before cooking)

Seasoning:
2tbsps cumin seeds
1 1/2tbsps crushed coriander seeds
2tbsps garam masala
1tbsp turmeric
1tbsp coriander powder
1tbsp salt
A little pepper

■ *Preparation*

1. Drain lentils and add new water, then simmer for twenty to thirty minutes, stirring occasionally.
2. Finely chop four onions. Then roughly chop two onions and blend these

for a couple of seconds until they turn into a thick paste – don't do it for too long or they will be completely liquid.

3. Throw all the onions, cumin seeds and crushed coriander seeds into a large heavy bottom pan and fry on a medium-high heat with ghee or olive oil until they start to brown.
4. Meanwhile blend the chilis, ginger and garlic into a fine paste.
5. Then mix the spices in a cup.
6. Once the onions are nice and soft and brown turn the heat down, add the paste and gently fry for ten minutes, stirring regularly. If the mixture gets too thick add a bit of water.
7. Add the spices and turn the heat up allowing the dal to bubble away for about ten minutes. Stir constantly so it doesn't stick. Add a little water if necessary.
8. By now, the cooked lentils should now be soft and a bit mushy. If not boil for a little longer and turn the heat right down on the onion mix.
9. Add the lentils, including any remaining liquid, to the onion mixture and stir well. Adjust the heat so that the dal simmers – you might need to add more water if it's still too thick. Reduce the dal for at least half an hour and up to an hour depending on how thick you want it to be stirring regularly.
10. Serve with rice or naan.

Morocco sits on the northwest coast of Africa, which is why its food contributes to the Mediterranean diet. Mainly influenced by Spain years ago, it produces fruits like orange, melons and tomatoes and vegetables such as potatoes and peppers. The Moroccan diet is rich in fish and seafood and some native ingredients including lemons, olives, almonds, figs and dates. A dish that has influenced other cultures is the famous cous cous, which is made from fine grains of wheat called semolina, and is usually served with vegetables, meat (except pork) and seafood. Another popular healthy dish that I have the pleasure of tasting whilst there is tajine. Tajine is a stew and I have included a great recipe for you to try.

Chicken tajine with almonds and prunes

Tajines, from North Africa, are delicious slow-cooked stews or meat and vegetables, served with cous cous as the carbohydrate. This recipe comes from Morocco where cooking with fruits such as lemons, olives, figs and dates is popular.

Ingredients

4 skinless, boneless chicken breasts
2tbsps olive oil
1tsp salt
1/2tsp ground black pepper
1tsp powdered cinnamon
1/4tsp powdered ginger
1/2tsp powdered saffron (optional)
3 short cinnamon sticksolive oil for frying
2 large onions
1 strip lemon peel
1lb dried prunes
Blanched almonds to garnish
Fresh watercress or mint

■ *Preparation*

1. Combine the oil and ground spices in a large bowl.
2. Cut the chicken into cubes and chop the onion. Add the chicken and onion to the bowl, combine well and leave to stand for thirty minutes.
3. Heat a small amount of olive oil in a large skillet, add the chicken and cook until golden brown.
4. Add the rest of the marinade and enough water to cover and then simmer until the chicken is tender – around thirty minutes.
5. While the chicken is cooking, put the prunes in a small saucepan, cover with water and bring the water to a boil. Remove the pan from the heat and let them stand for twenty minutes.
6. Drain the prunes, return them to the pan, and ladle a little liquid from the meat pan over the prunes. Simmer the prunes again for around five minutes then add the lemon peel and cinnamon sticks.
7. Plate up the meat and add the prunes to the meat Pour the sauce from the prunes over the meat and prunes.
8. While you are doing this set the rest of the liquid from the meat to reduce by half and pour over the meat and prunes.
9. Brown the almonds in a frying pan and use these and the watercress or mint to garnish.
10. Serve with brown rice or cous cous.

Ratatouille

Despite a cuisine that might lead you to think otherwise, the French diet is very healthy. Possibly, in part, because they have kept to traditional ways of preparing food and eating and haven't succumbed to processed food in the way we have.

They control their portion sizes to stop overeating and sit down at the table instead of snacking on the go as we do.

Ratatouille is a Provençale dish of stewed summer vegetables. This is delicious with grilled meats or on its own, with freshly baked bread to mop up the juices.

Ingredients

- **2 large-ish aubergines**
- **4 small courgettes**
- **4 large tomatoes – the vine-ripened ones work best as they have more flavour (don't use tinned).**
- **5 tbsps olive oil**
- **A small handful of basil**
- **I onion, peeled and thinly sliced**
- **3 crushed cloves of garlic**
- **I tbsp red wine vinegar**
- **I tsp sugar**

Preparation

1. Cut the aubergines and courgettes into inch cubes. Then deseed the peppers and cut into small chunks.
2. Skin the tomatoes by scoring the skin with a cross and immersing in boiling water for thirty seconds. Remove and plunge into cold water before peeling the skin away. Deseed the tomatoes and roughly chop the flesh.
3. Heat two tablespoons of olive oil in a pan and fry the aubergines for around five minutes until soft and brown. Then do the same for the courgettes in another tablespoon of oil and again for the peppers. Don't worry if they are still a bit hard.
4. Fry the onion in more olive oil for five minutes before adding the garlic. Fry for another minute before adding the vinegar, sugar, tomatoes and half the basil. Add the aubergines, courgettes and peppers, season and cook for another five minutes. Serve garnished with the remaining basil.

I am now thinking how amazing our diets and lifestyles could be if we introduced foods from around the world into our lives. Most of the ingredients for these foods are readily available in supermarkets and delis, so your challenge is to turn healthy eating into an adventure and learn to cook these delicious meals. I used to be a fussy eater, but once you have passed the first hurdle of trying new cuisines then, like me, there'll be no stopping you. So now my next chapter is on the superfoods that may be beneficial to you in more ways than you think.

CHAPTER 6

SUPERFOODS

'Food is the best medicine.'

Ann Wigmore

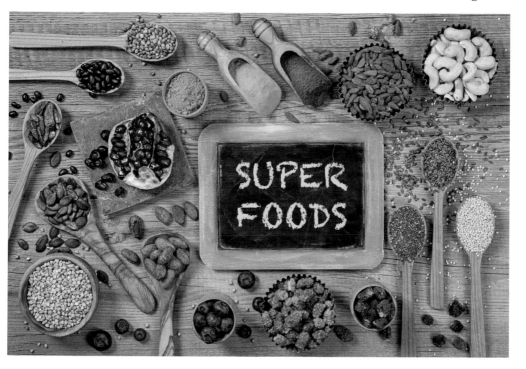

How many times do you hear 'you are what you eat'? The benefits of healthy eating, such as preventing heart attacks, strokes, cancers, diabetes and, of course, managing your weight, have already been covered so this chapter will look in more depth at a number of foods that have been singled out as superfoods and ask whether they really are superfood or super fad!

Superfoods are those that are said to keep our bodies from illness, nutritional deficiencies and threats of obesity. There is no technical definition for the term superfood, but the word is typically associated with foods that offer multiple benefits for the body without a high amount of fat and calories accompanying them. Every food labelled as superfood needs to be able to back up its claim with science. In actual fact producers often fund their own scientific studies to back certain claims.

The concern is that people will think eating one of these foods will offset the results of bad eating, when it is more complicated than that. To reap any benefits of superfoods, you need to eat them regularly as part of a balanced 'super diet' and not just to make up for eating a takeaway.

The Mediterranean diet we have already looked at is a good example as it includes lots of fruit and veg, olive oil, beans and pulses but is low on meat and dairy.

Examples of superfoods include:		
Beetroot	Blueberries	Broccoli
Chocolate	Garlic	Goji berries
Green tea	Oily fish	Pomegranate juice
Quinoa	Wheatgrass	

Broccoli

My uncle once told me that broccoli (and cauliflower) were both good for the mind as they looked like brains! I used to laugh but in actual fact I think he is right. Broccoli is the bestselling green vegetable in the UK and not only is it low in carbs, but it is also full of vitamins and fibre. It also contains high levels of cyanohydroxybutene; a substance which naturally replenishes the body's supply of glutathione, which people believe has some anti-cancer properties. Nothing has yet been proved but a study done by Dr Robert Thomas in Bedford Hospital highlighted one of his patients who believed that it helped him beat prostate cancer. The patient was on chemotherapy which was not working and his tumour weres getting bigger, so he decided to eat broccoli soup each day and when the results came back it showed the tumours had shrunk. Although there are many medical studies still to confirm this, it can't do any harm to eat it. Broccoli encourages healthy digestion and can aid in detoxification. It is also full of antioxidants that help limit the effects of free radical damage. Broccoli is also the perfect ingredient to accompany fish, meat or even put in a pasta or stir fry – it's even delicious in a soup so broccoli gets the thumbs up from me.

Green tea

This has been used in Chinese traditional medicine for centuries to relieve everything from depression to headaches. Green tea is full of antioxidants and contains vitamin B, folic acid and potassium. So where does it stand with weight-loss? Well, it's healthier than drinking a sugary drink or a coffee with three sugars! It is claimed that the antioxidants, catechin and caffeine, found in green tea may have a role in helping the body burn more calories so causing faster weight-loss, though at present there is no scientific evidence for this. I do believe that drinking it would be a benefit because of the antioxidants present.

If you are a big tea drinker, try switching to green tea which, since it is taken without milk or sugar, could save you thousands of calories a year.

Kale

I will be honest, I had never heard of kale up until a few years ago! I know: naughty me, however now I eat it lots. I use it as a vegetable with my Sunday dinners, in my stir fries and even in salad. Kale is rich in nutrients and helps to support bone, hair and skin health. These benefits also stretch to those with diabetes as it is claimed it can stabilise their blood sugar levels as well as balance blood pressure and studies are possibly developing a link to kale protecting against cancer. Low in calories and dense in nutrients, kale has a super effect on the human body and as well as being delicious I would recommend this leafy green to anyone.

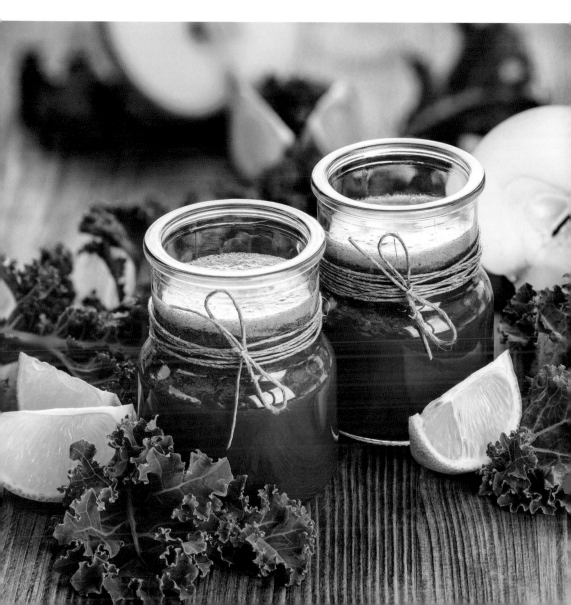

Sweet potato

It looks like carrots and in my opinion it tastes like carrots and turnips and I cannot get enough of it. You can mash it, bake it and even make sweet potato wedges! It's the beta carotene that gives this vegetable its orange colour which is the best part. These lovely potatoes are not only packed with nutrients their Vitamin C content is 2,000 times higher than a regular potato.

Wheatgrass

The idea that wheatgrass has super-beneficial properties has been around since the 1930s when US chemist Charles Schnabel inspired a body of scientific research. Wheatgrass contains chlorophyll that is said to boost the production of haemoglobin in the body. However, a dietician and spokesperson for BDA, Alison Hornby, has said that there is no real evidence for the claims that wheatgrass is better than other fruits and vegetables in terms of nutrition. Many juicing bars now sell shots of wheatgrass or add them to smoothies and claims have been made that one shot is equal to having your five a day, but there are no studies to support this. I can't see that there'd be any harm in having a shot as part of your five a day.

Quinoa

Quinoa is a full protein, high in fibre and (the best thing) it's gluten free. So how can this help with weight-loss? With only 222 calories per serving and a low glycaemic index, it is perfect. A low glycaemic index means it is digested more slowly by your body, leaving you feeling fuller for longer. A study at the University of Milan in 2005 backs this up. It found that quinoa was effective at controlling appetite and the participants consumed less food throughout the day. The study goes on to recommend quinoa as a food for dieters due to its high protein and low calorie nutritional profile. The best thing about this food is that it can be easily incorporated into your daily diet. Try new recipes using it and taste the delicious results. I love quinoa as it gives me a sense of fullness once I have eaten it and keeps me feeing full for longer than if I ate bacon on toast for breakfast! Below are breakfast, lunch and dinner recipes which contain quinoa and are easy to make at home.

BREAKFAST

Spiced chai quinoa

Ingredients

- I cup quinoa
- 2 cups milk – skimmed, almond, rice or soya depending on taste
- I large egg white
- I 1/2tbsps brown sugar, unpacked
- 1/4tsp pure vanilla extract
- 1/4tsp ground cardamom
- 1/4tsp ground cinnamon
- 1/4tsp ground ginger
- 1/4tsp nutmeg
- 2 dashes ground cloves

Preparation

1. Bring milk to a full simmer in a small saucepan. Add quinoa, return to a simmer and reduce heat to the lowest setting. Cover, leaving a tiny crack for steam to escape, and simmer until about two-thirds of the milk has been absorbed – about fifteen minutes.
2. Remove from heat and stir in the egg white, brown sugar and spices. Return pan to stove, covering again with a tiny crack for steam to escape, and continue to cook on low until almost all the milk has been absorbed – about five minutes.

LUNCH

Kale, quinoa and cherry salad

Ingredients

- 3tbsps extra-virgin olive oil
- 3tbsps cider vinegar
- 1/4tsp black pepper
- I 1/2 packets baby kale
- I 1/2 packets pre-cooked quinoa and brown rice mixed
- 3/4 cup fresh sweet cherries, pitted and halved
- 1/3 cup chopped fresh flat-leaf parsley
- 1/3 cup thinly sliced shallots
- I 14oz (400g) can unsalted chickpeas, rinsed and drained
- 1/2 cup of goat cheese, crumbled

■ *Preparation*

1. Combine ingredients into a bowl and stir for a refreshing salad. Add in olive oil and cider vinegar to taste, along with grind of black pepper to season.

DINNER

Quinoa and chickpea burgers

Ingredients

1/2 cup white quinoa
1 cup low-sodium vegetable broth
2 small slices wholewheat bread
14oz (400g) can chickpeas (drained and rinsed)
1 large egg
1 tspn cumin
1 small red chili
1 tbsp vegetable oil

■ *Preparation*

1. Put the quinoa and broth into a saucepan, bring to a boil on medium heat, reduce the heat and cover until the broth has been absorbed – around fifteen minutes.
2. Blitz the bread into fine breadcrumbs. Add the chickpeas, quinoa, egg, cumin and chili and blitz until the mixture is finely chopped. Shape the ingredients into four small burgers and brush with a little oil and grill under a medium to high heat for around four minutes each side. Serve with salad or rustle up some sweet potato wedges to go alongside.

Coconut oil

I have a confession to make: I love it so much I even put it on my face and in my hair as it makes a brilliant moisturiser and conditioner. It has also been linked to prevention of Alzheimer's and to boosting immunity. But how could it help with weight-loss? Coconut oil is easy to digest and it helps with the healthy functioning of the thyroid and endocrine system. Furthermore, it is said to increase the body's metabolic rate, thereby burning more energy and helping obese and overweight people lose weight. People who use coconut oil every day actually have a lower rate of heart diseae. Short-term studies have shown that it might also be effective in reducing hunger, since the men in the studies were seen to eat fewer calories after consuming coconut oil. If this is correct it may positively affect body weight over the long-term. I like to use coconut oil as an alternative to cooking oil as not only is better in health terms but also adds a unique flavour to my meat. I also add a teaspoon to smoothies for additional flavour and goodness. Try it and see what it can do for you.

Buckwheat

This gluten-free alternative to grains contains essential nutrients, healthy fat, vitamins and minerals, soluble and insoluble fibre and protein. It is possibly the world's healthiest food. Buckwheat is not a grain and it's nothing to do with wheat. It is actually a fruit seed. As a great healthy carbohydrate containing resistant fibre which is known to lower blood sugar levels and so help manage diabetes, it supports weight-loss and prevents IBS. A study published in *The American Journal of Clinical Nutrition* showed that eating 100g of buckwheat per day promoted healthy cholesterol levels. Buckwheat flour and pasta are great alternatives to refined pastas and baking goods. You can easily incorporate this into breakfast, lunch or dinner by using buckwheat instead of oats to make porridge or instead of rice to make risotto. Either way this is definitely worth a try.

Turmeric

Possibly the king of superfoods turmeric is best known as a curry spice, however its root is also used in medicine for arthritis, stomach pain, jaundice and bronchitis. Although this spice does not have any scientific evidence behind it to say that it helps with weight-loss, it is a superfood and it is used traditionally to

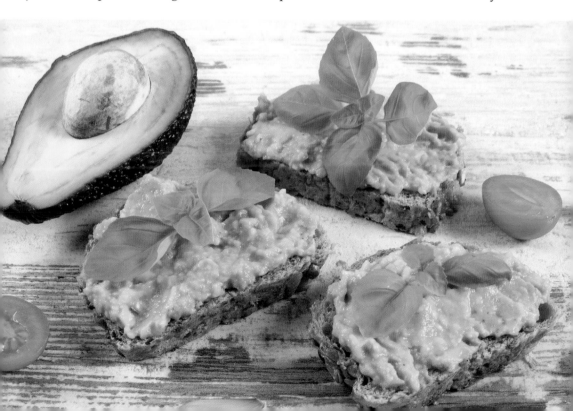

help with indigestion and its detoxifying properties may help cleanse the liver, enabling it to function more efficiently.

Avocado

Not only are avocados delicious, but they contain twenty different vitamins and minerals including vitamin K, vitamin C, folic acid and potassium. They also contain antioxidants and nutrients called lutein and zeaxanthin which have been proven to be important for eye health. It contains a monosaturated fat called oleic acid, which is associated with the reduction of low-density lipoprotein (LDL) or bad cholesterol. High levels of LDL can lead to diabetes mellitus. A recent article in *The Daily Telegraph* stated; a study in The *Journal of the American Association* has backed up the avocado's all-round awesomeness by showing that a group of overweight or obese patients who ate a moderate-fat diet including one avocado a day had significantly less LDL than people who ate the same diet but without the avocado. Not only that, but patients on the avocado diet also showed lower total cholesterol and levels of triglycerides (fat in the blood).

So is there anything actually wrong with this fruit? As it is also high in fibre, low in calories and low in carbs it is also great for weight-loss. It is versatile too: you can have it in a smoothie, spread it on toast, have it with some asparagus or prawns or make guacamole. Check out some of the recipes below.

Poached egg and avocado

Ingredients

1 avocado
2 eggs

■ *Preparation*

1. Bring 2-3 inches of water to a simmer in a pan. Separate the egg yolks from the whites and gently place the yolks into the water to poach. Cook for around a minute.
2. While the eggs are poaching, slice an avocado in half and remove the stone.
3. Remove each egg from the water and place in the avocado, use black pepper to season.

Mashed avocado and chickpea salad

Ingredients

1 avocado
1/2 lemon
A dollop of tahini
14oz (400g) can of chickpeas, rinsed and drained

1/2 cucumber, diced
2 stalks celery, chopped
I large carrot, chopped
2tbsps fresh dill
3tbsps salted sunflower seeds
2 wholegrain muffins
8 cherry tomatoes, halved

■ *Preparation*

1. Add the avocado, tahini, juice from half a lemon and chickpeas to a bowl. Using a fork or potato masher, mash these ingredients together.
2. Add the cucumber, celery, carrot, dill and sunflower seeds, and mix to combine. Season with pepper.
3. Serve the mixture on top of half a toasted English wholegrain muffin, top with four slices of cherry tomatoes.

Avocado, asparagus and sugar-snap pasta

Ingredients

I lb (460g) asparagus, ends trimmed and cut into 2-inch lengths
I lb (460g) sugar-snap peas, strings removed
I lb (460g) whole meal pasta
2 cloves garlic, minced
I avocado, halved, pitted, peeled, and cut into half-inch chunks
1/2 cup chopped fresh mint, parsley, or basil

■ *Preparation*

1. Cook the asparagus until bright green in a pan of boiling water for around two minutes. Add the sugar-snap peas and cook for another thirty seconds. Scoop out vegetables and put into a bowl.
2. Return water to a boil, add pasta and cook until al dente. Drain, reserving one cup of pasta water; set pasta aside in a colander.
3. In pasta pot add the asparagus, sugar-snap peas, and garlic and drizzle a little olive oil. Cook, tossing, until vegetables are also al dente. Add remaining ingredients and serve.

Water

Not really a superfood but probably the single most important thing you can put in your body. People often think that too much water is bad for us as they believe it causes bloating. However, it also helps flush toxins from your body, keeps you regular and its rehydrating properties help you look younger and healthier.

Exercising and a healthy diet is the best way to get rid of any water retention and remember that it might not be the water that's causing the problem, it could be wheat, medical conditions, dietary conditions, high salt intake and our body's reaction to hot weather. If you feel your stomach is bloating quite frequently then speak to your GP to establish if there is an no underlying cause.

Detox Water and infused water

Lemon slices in water is the homemade version of detox water. Now we can add almost anything to water to keep us hydrated. It's enjoyable and stimulating for the taste buds and the eyes. If you don't like drinking water this is the perfect way to enhance this free drink. As an added bonus, infused water has the sweet fruit flavours of fruit juice but without the extra calories or sugar. However, this is not true for the ones you buy in supermarkets so stay away from these and make your own at home.

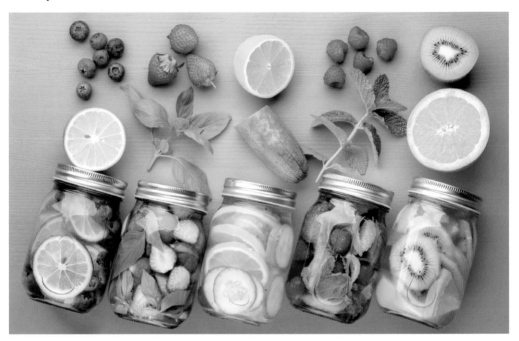

Here are some of my favourites!

Lemon and lime infusion – add half a lemon and half a lime and some chunks of orange to 2 litres of water

Tummy boost – add chunks of pineapple, add ginger and mint to 2 litres of water for a digestive superhero.

The antioxidant A team – half a cup each of strawberries, blueberries and blackberries added to 2 litres of water makes this a super delicious skin-plumping drink.

Bloating banished – add half a lemon, five slices of cucumber, ginger and mint to 2 litres of water and drink to help with stomach bloating.

Calm cravings – dding slices of apple and some cinnamon to 2 litres of water can help beat cravings. Delicious.

Watermelon wonder – simply add four slices of watermelon with some mint and 2 litres of water for a thirst-quenching drink.

Orange and blueberry – high in vitamin C this drink is ideal for those summer nights or even when you have been to the gym to keep you hydrated! Simply add four slices of orange and half a cup of blueberries to 2 litres of water.

Any of these will help on your weight-loss journey rather than drinking sugary drinks that are high in calories and contain bad sugar! You could add anything to water and make it taste amazing, you should leave the water to steep for at least two hours but it will last for two days, add ice for a truly refreshing drink and edible flowers to impress your guests.

Almost as good, though slightly higher in sugar, is adding your favourite fruit juice into sparkling water and making a juice spritzer. It's refreshing and a perfect summer alternative to wine spritzers. You could add half your favourite fresh juice and half sparkling water or sparkling water and a splash of cordial. Remember to check the sugar content though.

Now we have covered superfoods, we need to look at our shopping habits and how these can in fact affect us. How many of you go to the supermarket for a one-stop shop that includes not only healthy food but also a trip to the sweet and crisp aisles? Preparation before you leave the house is vital! Pre-plan your meals for the week then make a shopping list and ONLY BUY THOSE INGREDIENTS!

How to shop

I used to dread food shopping as it really was a chore, but now I love visiting different shops and thinking up new recipes. I also look out for local farmers' markets as I adore fresh produce and even though supermarkets are great, I enjoy local shops, particularly the butcher's. Call me old fashioned but I believe you can taste the difference in the butcher's meat. Shopping online is a great way too, though I prefer to get inspiration from the ingredients in front of me.

Loading up your trolley with healthy ingredients will not break your usual weekly budget and you will probably find after reading the food preparation section that you may actually save money as you are not wasting food! Compare the prices and take advantage of any multi-buy offers and also check the use-by dates! Frozen fruit, veg and fish will all last longer than a ready meal that needs to be eaten within three days of purchase. Think SMART. Here are some tips of food to avoid and foods you can swap.

Foods to avoid

Processed foods including processed meats and ready meals
Full fat milk and yogurts containing sugar
White bread, pasta and rice
Butter and cheese
Chips, wedges
Sweets, chocolate
Prepared desserts
Crisps
Savoury snacks
Fizzy drinks

Foods to buy

Fresh fruit and veggies
Chicken and turkey
Fish – white or oily
Semi-skimmed milk or skimmed
Wholegrain bread
Brown rice
Wholewheat pasta and noodles
Nuts and seeds
Pulses
Tinned fruit
Frozen fruit and vegetables
Bottles of water
Fresh fruit juice
Dried fruit

In the supermarket

- Choose natural, unprocessed ingredients, for example, oats, fruits and veggies, clean-cut meats and fish and brown rice.

- Do not choose foods which have sugar, diary or wheat as a main ingredient.

- Check the sugar content of the products you are buying.

- Foods that need advertising on TV are often not the best foods to be eating. Fresh food sells itself and does not need advertising.

- Choose foods that do not carry health claims such as 'low fat', 'sugar free' or 'zero calorie'. These can be the worst type of foods if you are trying to lose weight as they can be full of hidden calories.

- Foods labelled 'one of your five a day' are quite often misleading. Take care that an item really is one of your five a day. Some fruit juices and 'healthy' snack bars can be the calorie equivalent of eating a cake.

- Instant or fried foods along with readymade meals should be avoided, along with condiments, which should be used carefully. Sauces are often full of those bad fats and sugars so why not try making your own? Who knows, you could create a masterpiece.

- Think about going to markets and local shops as they are often the best way to discover new and healthy foods.

Use the traffic light system printed on packaging to show if foods are high in fat, salt and sugar! It is not an ideal system but it is helpful to those who are watching their weight or wanting to cut down something in particular.

Red = high – eat occasionally

Amber = medium – eat some of the time

Green = low – eat most of the time

Check the ingredient list! If the food you're trying to avoid shows up at the top of the list, then AVOID it.

I hope these tips will help you. I try to avoid buying processed foods as much as possible not just because of the calories, but also the health disadvantages. Now we have gone through the food we should be buying and the ones we could be eliminating, let us see some delightful recipes and snacks that we could try cooking as part of our plan.

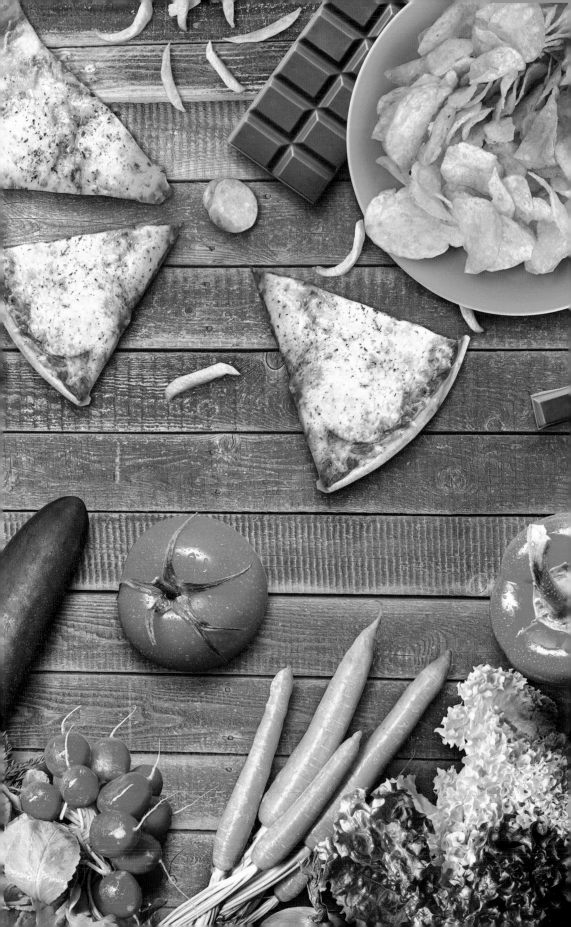

Chapter 7
Healthy Recipes and Food Swaps

'You don't have to eat less;

you just have to eat right'

Have you ever found yourself sneaking back to delicious unhealthy foods? Our challenge is to make the healthy stuff taste even better. We need to retrain our taste buds and this may seem daunting but healthy food can be made into fabulously appetising meals and snacks. Hopefully this chapter, full of recipes and food swaps, will help you create some new recipes for your shopping list and weekly menus. It also includes a list of foods and their calories to help you put together a balanced meal. This chapter has been my favourite to write as I love cooking and trying out different recipes. I am really excited to share some of my favourite dishes with help from a friend who is also a chef. I hope this will give you some insight into the ways you can approach a new healthier lifestyle and become excited about good foods.

Let us first talk about sauces. These are often high in sugar and fat but we often smother our food with them to make it taste better. People assume diet foods are bland and boring. Dry salads, dry chicken breasts or plain fish and bowls of steamed veggies don't really sound very appealing and if you don't enjoy your food you're unlikely to stick to your diet. The good news is that you can spice things up a little – fresh or dried herbs and spices are tasty and calorie free. Some sauces are also low-calorie with no sugar or fat so you needn't worry about them wrecking your diet.

Hot sauces

Hot sauces are generally very low in calories, as they're based around low-calorie ingredients; chillies, hot peppers, tomatoes and water. Hot sauces are a good addition to your diet as they're far lower in calories than ketchup or prepared pasta sauces. Avoid sweet chilli sauce however, as this contains high amounts of sugar.

Salsa

Salsa is a healthy, low-calorie dip. Salsa is predominantly tomato-based, with just onion, peppers and spices added. Look for low-sugar, low-salt salsas with no additives, or make your own by mixing tomatoes with other vegetables, lemon or lime juice and hot sauce or chillies. The advantage of doing this is that you control exactly what goes into your salsa and can make it as spicy or as mild as you wish to – if you are like me, mine would the mildest you can get!

Salad dressings

Store-bought salad dressings can be calorie bombs, loaded with sugar, salt and fat. Making your own is a far healthier option by combining olive oil with vinegar or lemon juice, or making a low-calorie creamy dressing with fat-free Greek yogurt, grated ginger, minced garlic, low-sodium soy sauce, olive oil and lemon juice. Making your own means you can keep track of exactly what goes into your dressing and you are also experimenting with new flavours to suit your needs and desires.

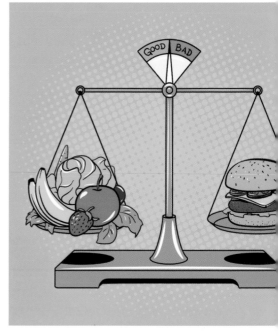

Sweet sauces

When you feel the need for something sweet, make a coulis using fruit to satisfy your craving rather than reaching for the sweet jar. Take a mix of fruits and blitz them in a blender, adding a little water if needed. Blackberries, strawberries and blueberries are perfect for this or you could try using peanut butter and honey for different flavours.

Now we have looked at sauce swaps let us try looking at food swaps and how to change the way we think about the foods we eat.

Food swaps

Simple food swaps could make a profound difference in your daily diet. Are you a bread lover? Do you have a sweet tooth? Are you a lover of cheese? I will look at other alternatives that may benefit you and also foods that can help beat those cravings.

Whole milk	>	Coconut milk / almond milk / soy milk / skimmed
Tea/coffee	>	Flavoured herbal teas / Green tea
Sugary drinks	>	Flavoured fruit water
Cordial	>	Coconut water
Sugary cereals	>	Muesli / porridge
White bread	>	Wholegrain bread
Biscuits	>	Oatcakes
Cream cheese	>	Feta cheese
Cream	>	Crème fraîche
Philadelphia cheese	>	Hummus
Chips	>	Sweet potato wedges
Crisps	>	Nuts, sunflower seeds
Potatoes	>	Sweet potato
Mashed potato	>	Mashed cauliflower or broccoli
Processed meats	>	Fresh meat from deli
Red meat	>	Chicken / turkey / pork
Sausages	>	Homemade meatballs
Sauces	>	Create your own. For example, tomato sauce can be easily made from chopped tomatoes
Fried eggs	>	Poached, boiled or scrambled egg
Butter	>	Apple sauce
Cooking oil	>	Olive oil / coconut oil
Salted nuts	>	Unsalted nuts (pistachios, almond, cashew)
Sweets	>	Unsalted popcorn
Salt	>	Herbs and spices
Desserts	>	Fruit salad / poached pears

Drinks

Don't become confused. We discussed earlier how water is the best drink if you want to be healthy but you don't have to drink it neat or flavoured with fruit. You can also get it from tea, coffee and juice. As said before sugary drinks are technically classed as part of the fluid intake but are not as advised due to their high sugar content. The same goes for energy drinks. Many people drink energy drinks for a boost when tired, however it is not advised. These can be highly addictive and not to mention high in sugar. In the EU, it is estimated that 30 per cent of adults and 68 per cent of young people drink energy drinks, with global sales estimated to be around $12 billion in 2012. Since energy drinks contain a variety of complicated ingredients with scientific names it is hard to keep track of what you're consuming. Warning labels are displayed on the packaging but there is a risk to children who are consuming them more frequently. Pubs and clubs now serve energy drinks mixed with alcohol, which can be dangerous. A study completed in Australia highlighted the risks from data collected over seven years. The list is in order of the most common to the least common;

1. Palpitations
2. Tremors / shaking
3. Agitation / shaking
4. Stomach upset
5. Chest pains
6. Dizziness
7. Tingling skin
8. Insomnia
9. Respiratory distress
10. Headaches

Caffeine is the biggest ingredient in these types of drinks and caffeine addiction can cause increased blood pressure, palpitations, increased urination, headaches, dizzy spells, nausea and fatigue. They are also high in sugars including high fructose corn syrup and can cause teeth decay, obesity and sugar addiction. In the media recently there have been reported deaths from people overdosing on energy drinks. I would avoid them especially if you are suffering from a medical condition: there are no long-term studies of effects of consuming energy drinks so it's impossible to know what they are doing to us.

Caffeine

Caffeine is a stimulant to the central nervous system, which is why we consume it to wake ourselves up and why coffee drinkers say it makes them alert and better able to concentrate. It is naturally found in certain leaves, beans and fruits of over sixty plants worldwide. Caffeine can also be produced synthetically and added to food, beverages, supplements and medications. It is addictive so if you choose to give it up, some of the withdrawal symptoms you may experience are headaches, fatigue, anxiety, irritability, depression and lack of concentration. It is recommended that you drink no more than three cups a day or that you go for one of the caffeine free coffees available.

Caffeine is also present in tea so if you are concerned about your intake you

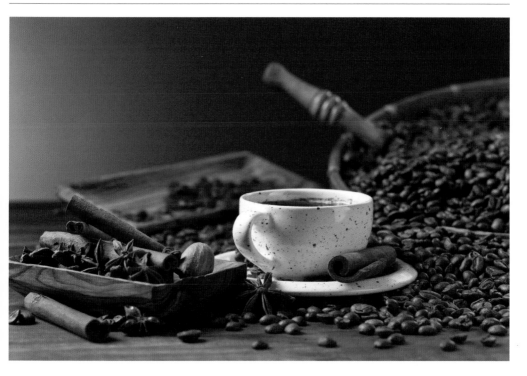

could try a caffeine free tea, or better still go for a herbal or fruit tea such as green tea, camomile, peppermint or red bush. Green tea, as discussed earlier, is believed to have health-boosting properties and aid with weight-loss. In my opinion, herbal and flavoured teas are more beneficial than fizzy drinks.

Caffeine and weight-loss.

Many of the supplements now state that caffeine is a 'fat burning' product and an 'appetite suppressant', but the research to support this is inconclusive as this report from the website Medicinenet shows: The scientific evidence about caffeine as a weight-control agent is mixed. In a study done to monitor the impact of a green tea-caffeine combination on weight-loss and maintenance, participants were divided into those who consume low levels of caffeine (<300mg/day) and high-caffeine consumers (>300mg/day). Weight-loss was significantly higher in the high-caffeine consumption group, but weight maintenance was higher in the low-caffeine consumption group. The conclusion was that the caffeine was related to greater weight-loss, higher thermogenesis, and fat oxidation, while the tea was responsible for the greater weight maintenance. Other studies have stated that caffeine actually contributes to weight gain due to the increasing stress hormones. It appears that caffeine's role in weight-loss is as inconclusive as the efficacy of the majority of weight-loss supplements on the market.

The US Food and Drug Administration (FDA) and the American Medical Association (AMA) classify a 'moderate intake' of caffeine as 'generally recognized as safe'. So like everything else caffeine is safe within moderation. However, I would not advise supplements which contain caffeine such as energy supplements or weight-loss pills.

Alcohol

Alcohol is often the biggest obstacle when it comes to losing weight. Beer drinkers should know that if they drink five pints a week, that comes to 44,200 calories over a year or the equivalent of consuming 221 doughnuts. Five pints of cider in one night is the equivalent of 1,020kcal, which is half a woman's daily calorie requirement. If you drink spirits with mixers then you are taking in the calories in these as well. Since drinking is associated with food and socialising you probably eat more too, either because you have a bottle of wine with your meal or because you eat before or after a big night out to line your stomach. I am almost certain the majority of people have a greasy fry up the next day to cure that hangover too. This may not sound much if you are an occasional drinker but if you have a lively social life that involves drinking every weekend, or you like a glass of wine or two in the evening, then you can see how this could create a spare tyre. And these are empty calories – there are no nutritional benefits in most forms of alcohol, though there is evidence that drinking red wine reduces the risk of heart disease and keeps bedbugs at bay – should this be a problem!

So how many calories are in alcoholic drinks. Here is a table you can see how a few drinks quickly add up

Alcoholic	Calories
Standard glass of wine (175ml)	125kcal
Pint of 5% proof lager	215kcal
50ml glass of cream liqueur	118kcal
Vodka and coke (175ml)	120kcal
Gin and tonic (single)	120kcal
Gin and slimline tonic (single)	56kcal
Dry cider (pint)	204kcal
Whisky and lemonade (175ml)	82kcal

How can we cut down? Let us take a look at various ways that may help you.

TIPS TO CUT DOWN

Stick to the recommended fourteen units per week, this way you know you are not overloading yourself. Next, eat healthy foods before you go out, don't drink on an empty stomach or you'll be craving snacks or greasy food on the way home! And your hangover will be much worse leading to bad eating the following day. Don't think that saving up your units allows you to go binge-drinking on the weekend – it doesn't. In fact, don't go binge drinking at all – it's bad for you in very many ways, not just in terms of weight gain. Stay away from buying rounds of drinks as you will end up consuming more – especially if those with you are drinking quickly. Alternately an alcoholic drink with a glass of water keeps you hydrated and reduces your intake and keeps you hydrated. A glass of fizzy water is easily disguised as a gin and tonic if you are worried about peer pressure. If you drink pints try cutting down to halves, swap cocktails for mocktails or strong drink for alcohol-free. Reducing your alcohol intake also reduces the risk of a hangover. Have a plan in place if you are determined to kick alcohol altogether: if you know you could be drinking then drive – it gives you the perfect excuse to stick to soft drinks. If you can't resist temptation then remove it altogether by doing something else instead: have a bath, start a new hobby, try a sport or exercise class, do a bit of DIY. Not only will you be healthier, you'll be financially better off too. You'll be shocked by how much money you spend on a night out. Put this money to one side and use it to treat yourself when you hit your weight targets. These are just few ideas I think will work if you are committed to starting a healthy change in life.

Drink plenty of water to stay hydrated. If you feel jaded the next day do some moderate exercise. This will sweat it out of you, fill you full of energy and clear your mind.

If you feel you need help with drinking contact a doctor or a local support group such as Alcoholics Anonymous who will talk to you in complete confidence.

Recipes

I am so excited to share some of these amazing healthy recipes, which everyone will enjoy. I hope you will try these out and find them as delicious as I do. I have made them simple and varied to give you an idea how delicious and enjoyable healthy eating can be. So even if you find cooking a chore, I think you will like these. I wish I could add more to this section, however I think that these recipes will be enough to give you the clean eating bug, then you can find more recipes on the internet or in books.

Food is essential to life, therefore make it good.

BREAKFAST

Egg soldiers with asparagus and prosciutto

This oh-so-simple recipe will have you jumping out of bed in the morning. It is quick and easy to prepare – within ten minutes you will have consumed one of your five a day plus some protein. It is great for a weekend brunch instead a full English breakfast.

Ingredients

    2 eggs
    4 slices of prosciutto
    8 asparagus spears

■ *Preparation*

1. Place the eggs into a pan of boiling water and simmer for four minutes until soft boiled. Remove from water and place in eggcups.
2. Meanwhile cut the prosciutto in half longways and wrap around the asparagus spears.
3. Place the wrapped asparagus spears under a medium-hot grill for four minutes, until the asparagus is tender and prosciutto is slightly crispy.
4. Cut the tops off your eggs and dip the asparagus into the yolk.

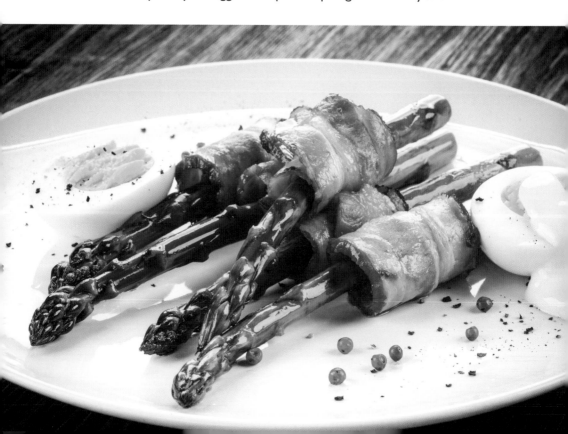

Poached eggs with grilled kipper

Great for anyone who loves kippers. This quick and easy recipe ensures you are starting your day with omega 3.

Ingredients

I egg
3oz (80g) spring greens
3.5oz (90g) of kipper fillets
Black pepper

Preparation

1. Boil water in a pan, stir with a spoon to create a swirl within the water and then crack the egg into the middle of it.
2. Turn the heat down and simmer for four minutes. Wilt the spring greens by placing them in a colander over the pan for the last minute of cooking time.
3. Grill the kippers for three to five minutes then drain the eggs and spring greens
4. Serve the poached egg on top of the kipper and spring greens and season with black pepper.

Walnut and salmon breakfast salad

You may think salad for breakfast is not quite right and if this really bothers you, try this dish as a tasty lunch. I am a lover for salad and could eat it throughout the day. This salad is not only delicious but quick and easy to prepare.

Ingredients

2 eggs
Bowl of fresh spinach
Smoked salmon
I sliced apple
Handful of walnuts
Extra virgin olive oil and balsamic vinegar to dress

Preparation

1. Bring saucepan of water to the boil.
2. Crack in two eggs and boil for one to two minutes until white.
3. Serve eggs on bed of spinach and smoked salmon.
4. Cover with apple, walnuts and dressing.

Granola with strawberries and orange

This yummy recipe makes enough to last a week saving you time in the morning.

Ingredients

14oz (400g) jumbo oats
Juice of 2 oranges plus zest of 1/2 an orange
1tsp ground cinnamon
2tbsp freeze-dried strawberries
1oz (25g) flaked almonds toasted
1oz (25g) mixed seeds (such as sunflower, pumpkin, sesame and linseed)

■   *Preparation*

1. Put 200g oats and 500ml water in a food processor and blend for one minute. Line a sieve and pour in the oat mixture. Leave to drip through for five minutes. Put this creamy liquid in a sealed jug and place in the fridge. It'll keep for three days.
2. Heat the oven to 200C/180C fan/gas 6 and line a baking tray with baking parchment. Put the orange juice into the saucepan and bring to the boil. Boil for five minutes or until the liquid has reduced by half, stirring occasionally. Mix the remaining oats with the orange zest and cinnamon. Remove the pan from the heat and stir the oat mixture into the juice. Spread over the tray in a thin layer and cook for ten to fifteen minutes. Leave to cool down in the tray.
3. Once the oat brittle has cooled, break into pieces and mix with the strawberries, flaked almonds and seeds. The granola can be kept for up to one week in a sealed storage box or jar. Serve in a bowl with the oat milk poured over the top.

SOUPS

Spring green special soup

This soup is super quick to prepare so you don't have any excuse about time with this one!

Ingredients

1tbsp olive oil
4 medium leeks (sliced)
1 litre low-salt stock
6 1/2oz (180g) soya beans (frozen are best)
6 1/2oz (180g) spring greens
6 spring onions
Black pepper and thyme to season

■ *Preparation*

1. Heat the olive oil in a large pan on a medium-low heat. Add the leeks and cook until soft.
2. Add the stock and bring to a boil. Add in the soya beans and cook for approximately two minutes.
3. Add the spring greens and cook for a further minute. Ladle into bowls.
4. Sprinkle the spring onions into each bowl and season to taste with pepper and thyme.

Sweet potato and coconut milk soup

I adore sweet potato and coconut milk so combining this is heaven. Fast and fabulous and what is better is you can make this last for a couple of days and the whole family will love it.

*Ingredients*_____

2tsp vegetable oil
I onion, diced
Itbsp finely chopped fresh ginger
Itbsp vegan Thai red curry paste
I 1/2lb (660g) sweet potatoes, diced
14oz (400ml) canned reduced-fat coconut milk
I litre vegan stock

■ *Preparation*

1. In a large saucepan, heat the oil over a medium-high heat. Add the onion and ginger and cook, stirring occasionally, for about five minutes until soft.
2. Add the curry paste and cook for a further minute while stirring. Add the sweet potatoes, coconut milk and stock and bring to the boil. Reduce the heat to medium and simmer for about twenty minutes or until the sweet potatoes are soft.
3. Purée the soup using a blender, food processor or hand-held blender. Return the soup to the heat and simmer. Serve and enjoy.

Watercress and asparagus soup

Did anyone else used to make watercress sandwiches in school? I did and watercress was not my favourite food! This little discovery completely changed my opinion.

Ingredients

32floz (900ml) vegetable stock
I small cauliflower, trimmed and chopped
12oz (350g) asparagus spears, chopped
4 spring onions
2oz (50g) watercress
Black pepper to taste

■ *Preparation*

1. Put the cauliflower in a large pan and bring to the boil. Add the asparagus and spring onions, bringing back to the boil and simmer for three minutes.
2. Remove from the boil and stir in the watercress and mint until wilted. Blend the soup in blender or use hand blender and then reheat and season with pepper.

Creating the ideal soup

As well as these recipes, here are some general tips on making soups. People think it's time-consuming but in half an hour you could have a healthy, nutritious meal for a family. If you have a slow cooker you can leave it all day. Soup freezes well, so try making double quantities and you'll have your own homemade ready-meals. All you need is a blender. Let me explain the tips I think will help you:

1. Choosing a type of fat

Your soup will probably need to start with some type of healthy fat like olive oil. This is to sauté any root vegetables or other initial ingredients. Choose whatever you have on hand that will mesh well with your flavours. I would choose olive oil for an Italian soup with a tomato base. If you are using butter, try not to use too much.

2. Choosing the base

What do you have on hand? Chicken, beef or fish stock? Tomato purée? Choose one. Stock mixed with tomato purée is lovely, as is stock with milk. Or even cream with tomato purée – though go steady on the cream or you won't lose any weight. You pick the flavours you want; it is your soup.

3. Choosing the meat

If you want meat, that is. You may be veggie. Choose whatever you like or whatever you have at home. You'll probably want this to match your base (beef with fish stock might not be such a great combination), but use what you have.

4. Choosing your veggies

Onion is a pretty standard veggie because it imparts so much flavour. Garlic, carrots, and celery are all good for soups too. There are also beans, spinach, kale, corn, and so on. Use whatever you have, and whatever you like! Potatoes make a good thickener if you want a creamy low-fat soup without the calories.

5. Choosing the seasoning

Sea salt and black pepper are your two most basic seasonings, so you will want to include them. Here are a few more popular seasonings – all add deliciousness with no extra calories.

Celery seed, marjoram, thyme, parsley, and sage go well with chicken. Marjoram, rosemary and thyme go well with beef. Basil, oregano or fennel can be a nice addition to tomato-based soups.Hot soups need chili powder and perhaps cumin. Creamy soups might benefit from a dash of parsley or thyme. Dream up any combination you like, soup does not have to be bland and boring! Taste and adjust as you go!

LUNCHES

There is no excuse for not preparing these quick lunches which are also ideal for work. It takes five minutes and they are really tasty.

Tuna Stuffed peppers - serves 2

Ingredients

- 2 red peppers
- 2 green peppers
- 4 tins of tuna
- 2tbsp of olive oil
- 1 red onion, chopped thinly

■ *Preparation*

1. Slice the top off the peppers and deseed them.
2. Mix together the tuna and olive oil.
3. Add in the red onion.
4. Pour the tuna and red onion into each of the stuffed peppers.

Cajun steak salad – serves 1

You don't have to avoid red meat all the time and I do love steak without the fat! I have mine medium and this speedy lunch takes only minutes to cook.

Ingredients

   1 head Romaine lettuce
   8 cherry tomatoes, cut in half
   1 cucumber, peeled and sliced
   1 roasted pepper cut into strips
   2 radishes, sliced any other salad vegetable you might feel like cajun spice seasoning piece of steak, fat removed

■ *Method*

1. Prepare salad in large bowl and set aside.
2. Sprinkle cajun spice mix over steak on both sides.
3. Heat oil in a griddle and cook steak to your liking.
4. Slice steak and place on top of salad.

Turkey lettuce boats – serves 2

Sounds intriguing? These little lettuce boats are not only filling but full of protein from the turkey. I love these clever little creations and they are super-fast to prepare too.

Ingredients

   4 iceberg lettuce leaves
   2 cooked turkey breasts, sliced
   1/2 cucumber, cut into long strips
   4 spring onions, cut into long strips
   250g hummuspaprika

■ *Preparation*

1. Place sliced turkey breast with cucumber, onion, hummus and a sprinkling of

paprika in lettuce leaf. Then wrap with another leaf to make a wrap. Repeat with remaining ingredients.

Takeaway style kebab – serves 2

Try a takeaway-style kebab but prepare it yourself. Yummy and not full of sauces and fat.

Ingredients

I pound of minced beef
I whole egg
I/2tsp black pepper
Itsp garlic powder
I/2tsp sea salt
I/2tsp chilli powder
Itbsp chives
4tbsp low fat Greek yogurt

■ *Preparation*

1. In a mixing bowl, blend the minced beef, egg (beaten), black pepper, sea salt, chilli powder, and I/2tsp garlic powder, shaping it into a loaf. It's best to use your hands for this.
2. Place it on a baking tray and cook in a pre-heated over for one hour twenty minutes, turning half way through so that it browns evenly.
3. Mix the yogurt, chives and I/2tsp garlic powder to form a garlic dip.
4. Once cooked thoroughly, slice it very thinly and serve with a side salad.

Salmon, broad bean and red lentil pasta

This is great for filling up on omega fats, fibre and protein and takes under fifteen minutes to create.

Ingredients

2 cups mixed salad leaves
3 spring onions, sliced
I/2 cup mangetout
I/2 cup broad beans
I/4 cucumber, diced
I/2 packet of red lentil pasta
Olive oil
Itsp lemon juice
Herbs

■ *Preparation*

1. Heat the grill to medium heat and line the grill with tin foil.
2. Place the salmon on top of foil and drizzle over some lemon and olive oil.
3. Grill for around fifteen minutes until it is cooked.
4. Once cool break the salmon into pieces,
5. Combine the rest of the ingredients into a small bowl.
6. Place the pasta into a pan of boiling water and cook until al dente.
7. Toss the pasta in herbs and olive oil then add the salmon and the rest of the ingredients. Serve with a salad.

Red onion and mixed peppers on toast

Ingredients

   2 peppers
   1 small red onion cut into thin wedges
   2tsp olive oil
   4 slices wholemeal bread
   125g low-fat mozzarella cheese sliced
   1 pinch ground black pepper

■ *Preparation*

1. Preheat the grill to medium.
2. Arrange the peppers on foil with the red onion. Sprinkle with the olive oil and grill until soft and lightly browned.
3. Toast the slices of bread and divide the peppers and onion between them. Arrange the mozzarella on top, return to the grill for one to two minutes, until the cheese has melted.
4. Serve with salad

Salads – they don't need to be boring

Salads do not need to be dull, plain or tasteless. You can add anything into a salad to make it delicious: meat, fish, veggies and even fruit but check out my few pointers to make you want to devour salad every day!

Cleaning the leaves

Simply rinse lettuce and salad ingredients under a tap, but to make sure you get the excess dirt off and ensure there are no more chemicals place them in a bowl full of water and rub gently. Ensure the salad is thoroughly dried. Washed salad can keep in the fridge for a few days, but it is better to clean it as you need it.

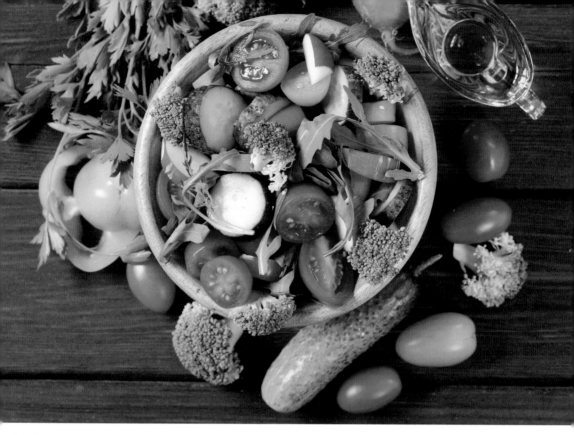

Add some salt

If you are making your own dressing of oil and vinegar season it to enhance the salad's flavour. Don't worry about eating too much salt as it'll only be a sprinkling. If you are worried go for a low-sodium salt instead.

Texture

Liven your salad up with by adding different textures, chefs say texture is everything when it comes to food so add a few nuts or a crumbly cheese to keep your tastebuds happy. Balance the flavours

The salad should have a range of flavours whether salty, spicy, sweet, acidic or bitter. Flavour will make the salad appetising and will inspire you to experiment with new combinations. Stay in season

Stay in season with the greens. Try kale and Brussels sprouts during winter and romaine lettuce during the spring and summer. This will stop things becoming boring. It'll save you money too as food bought in season is always cheaper.

Portion size

Since there are no calories in salads make sure you have as much as you need to feel full, or you will be hungry shortly after. Just go easy on the other ingredients such as fish or cheese, nuts or dressing as these are where the calories lurk.

Herbs and seasoning

Herbs and other seasonings are packed with flavour but have zero calories so you can use them to boost flavour. Use fresh ones in among the leaves or dried ones in your dressing. Edible flowers are a great way to make your salads look more colourful too

Dress the salad

A homemade vinaigrette of balsamic vinegar and olive oil is the obvious choice but try jazzing things up with flavoured oils and vinegars. Avocado and walnut oils or rice and fruit-infused vinegars are also great substitutes.

The main show

If you are serving an accompaniment to your salad – say a piece of grilled fish or meat make it look, and taste really appetising. Appealing food makes us want to eat it. Try unusual foods to finish off your salad – your friends will think you have become a chef overnight.

Check out these recipes I have put together for you.

Quinoa, feta & pomegranate salad – 4 servings

Ingredients

3tbsp extra virgin olive oil
7oz (200g) quinoa
7oz (200g) tenderstem broccoli
7oz (200g) feta cheese
2tbsp pumpkin seeds
I pomegranate seedsI large handful chopped parsley4 tomatoes, chopped
3 spring onions
3tbsp lemon juice

■ *Preparation*

1. Cook the quinoa according to the packet and leave to cool.
2. Meanwhile steam the broccoli and toast the pumpkins seeds in a small frying pan until crunchy.
3. Once the hot ingredients have cooled, stir together with feta, pomegranate, spring onions, herbs and tomatoes.
4. Drizzle with olive oil and lemon juice. Season with pepper.

Shrimp and orange salad – serves 2-3

Ingredients

10 1/2oz (300g) pack of free-range egg noodles
9oz (260g) pack cooked and peeled jumbo king prawns
2 oranges, peeled and segmented
3 1/2oz (100g) pack watercress
1 red onion sliced
3tbsp sweet chilli sauce
Juice of one lime
2 lettuces, leaves separated

■ *Preparation*

1. Toss together the noodles, prawns, orange segments, red onion and watercress.
2. Mix together the sweet chilli sauce and lime juice, pour over the noodle salad.
3. Arrange the lettuce leaves in a bowl and pile the noodle salad into the centre.

Celery and almond salad

Simple but sweet salad

Ingredients

1 head of celery (12-15 stalks), plus leaves
1 cup flaked almonds
1/4 cup olive oil
2 teaspoons lemon juice
1/4 cup roughly chopped parsley
salt and pepper

■ *Preparation*

1. Chop the celery stalks and leaves into bite-size pieces. Mix together with almonds.
2. Whisk together the olive oil, lemon juice, parsley, and a pinch of salt and pepper together in a small bowl. Pour the dressing on top of the celery and almonds and stir. Serve with grilled low-fat halloumi cheese.

Minty roast veg and hummus salad

Ingredients

4 parsnips, peeled and cut into wedges
4 carrots, cut into wedges
2tsp cumin seeds
14oz (400g) can chickpeas, drained
2tbsp olive oil
2tbsp clear honey
7oz (200g) pot hummus
2tbsp white wine vinegar
1 small bunch of mint leaves
7oz (200g) block feta cheese

Preparation

1. Heat oven to 180°C. Toss the parsnips, carrots and chickpeas with the oil, cumin seeds and some seasoning in a large roasting tin. Cook for thirty minutes, tossing halfway through cooking.

2. Drizzle over the honey, then return to the oven for around ten minutes.

3. Spread the hummus thinly over a large platter, or divide between four dinner plates. When the veg is ready, drizzle with the vinegar and toss together in the tin.

4. Tip the roasted vegetables on top of the hummus, scatter over the mint and cheese.

OMELETTE CHOICES

Omelettes are not only good for us but we can add almost anything we like to vary the flavours – they are perfect for breakfast, lunch or dinner! Also you only need a sprinkling of the filling so if you like cheese or smoked sausage, you'll love these. Here my top fifty ideas for omelette fillings:

1. Smoked salmon
2. Swiss cheese and tomatoes
3. Herbs
4. Spinach
5. Red peppers
6. Mushrooms, bell peppers and low-fat cheese
7. Jalapenos, spinach and bell pepper with salsa topping
8. Cheese, peppers, tomato and onion
9. Mushrooms
10. Tomatoes

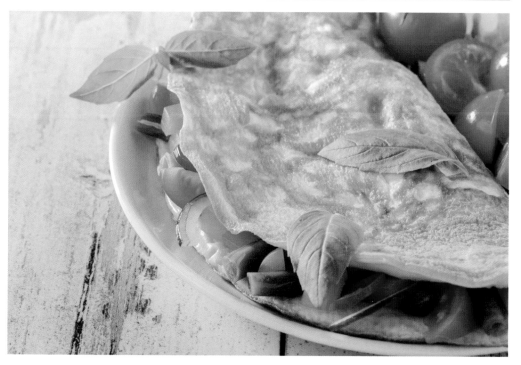

11. Crumbled grilled bacon, mushrooms, tomatoes and onion
12. Swiss cheese and turkey bacon
13. Spinach, onion, red pepper and feta
14. Spinach, tomatoes, onion and mushrooms
15. Spinach, bacon and feta
16. Asparagus and cheese
17. Spring onion, bacon and sour cream
18. Goat cheese, spinach and tomatoes
19. Peppers, onion, parsley, tomatoes, arugula or spinach, chili peppers and goat cheese
20. Spinach, mushrooms, prosciutto, olives,
21. artichokes, peppers, broccoli
22. Ham
23. Onion, sweet corn, pepper, cheese
24. Smoked haddock and parmesan
25. Crab and avocado
26. Chive, tomato and goat cheese
27. Smoked mozzarella, sun-dried tomato, basil pesto
28. Salmon and asparagus
29. Asparagus
30. Chorizo
31. Caramelized onion and spinach
32. Chillies and feta

33. Onions, jalapenos and cheese topped with salsa
34. Artichoke hearts sautéed with garlic and seasoned goat cheese
35. Turkey bacon and avocado
36. Basil, tomatoes, mozzarella
37. Spinach and nuts
38. Chicken and portabello mushrooms
39. Leeks and peppers with feta cheese
40. Salmon and asparagus with added spices
41. Chicken sausage, avocado and red onion
42. Spinach, garlic and low-fat cream cheese
43. Tuna and red onion
44. Green olives
45. Pancetta
46. Pancetta and feta
47. Mixed spices and chicken
48. Prawns
49. Smoked salmon and capers
50. Roast vegetables

MAIN COURSES

Do you ever feel it is too much of an effort to cook a meal or think that you don't have the time? The recipes below contain a variety of meals, some of which are simple and quick and some may take time but are well worth it as the end result is nutritious, cost effective a healthy way to lose weight. Remember that cooking can be enjoyable and you can make it by turning off the TV and talking to each other or by having friends over. You can use the internet for recipe ideas, or buy a new healthy cook book as a reward for losing weight. Take a look at these recipes for some inspiration.

Fish stew

If you are a lover of fish, then you will love this dish.

Ingredients

1 tbsp olive oil
1 cup chopped onion
1/4 cup chopped celery
1 tsp chili powder
1 1/2 cups frozen whole kernel corn
1 tbsp Worcestershire sauce
1 can no-salt-added diced tomatoes

2 cups water
1 1/2lb (680g) cod, cut into bite size pieces (or any white fish fillets)
1/4 cup chopped parsley
salt and pepper for seasoning

Preparation

1. Heat oil in a pan over a medium to high heat.
2. Add onion, celery and chili powder and sauté for three minutes or until tender.
3. Stir in the corn, Worcestershire sauce, diced tomatoes and water and cook for a further ten minutes.
4. Add the fish, and cook for five minutes or until the fish is done.
5. Taste and season with salt and pepper to taste.
6. Stir in the parsley and serve.

Chicken and spinach curry – serves 4

If you a curry lover, then this recipe is for you. You can make this spicy or mild depending on your taste buds.

Ingredients

1tsp olive oil
17oz (480g) chicken breasts, diced
2 cloves garlic, crushed
2tsp coriander
2tsp cumin
2tsp turmeric
1tsp chilli powder
1 tin chopped tomatoes
3 1/2floz (100ml) low-salt chicken stock
6oz (160g) baby spinach
To serve
2 cups brown rice

Preparation

1. Heat the olive oil into a frying pan on a medium-low heat. Add the chicken and fry until browned.
2. Add in the ginger, garlic and spices and stir for around one minute.
3. Add in the tomatoes and the stock and simmer for five minutes until it is slightly reduced.
4. Cook the rice according to the packet instructions.
5. Stir the spinach into the chicken curry just before serving.
6. Put the rice onto a plate and then add the curry.

Kale and sprout stir fry – serves 2

As a lover of kale, this is a favourite of my mine. Since stir-fry is so versatile you can add all kind of vegetables, so don't be afraid to experiment. Use enchanting colours which makes it look even more appetising and don't forget to use spices to create your own flavours.

Ingredients

8oz soba noodles
8tsp sesame oil
7oz (200g) kale
8 Brussels sprouts
1 clove garlic
1tbsp brown rice wine vinegar
1tsp soy sauce
1tbsp sesame seeds
1 pinch of red chilli flakes

■ *Preparation*

1. Cook the soba noodles according to the packet instructions. Drain and toss with three teaspoons of the sesame oil.
2. While the noodles are cooking, prepare the veggies. Wash and dry the kale and put the dry leaves into the bowl. Add two teaspoons of the sesame oil and rub into the kale to soften it.
3. Peel and slice the Brussels sprouts as thinly as possible. Cut the slices into slivers, then toss with the kale.
4. Crush the garlic and whisk into the rice vinegar, then add the remaining three teaspoons of sesame oil and the soy sauce. Whisk until you have a smooth dressing. Pour over the kale and Brussels sprouts. Add the cooked noodles, sesame seeds, and red chilli flakes.

Squash risotto – 4 servings

A delicious warming dish for autumn.

Ingredients

450g butternut squash
2 14oz (400g) tins chickpeas
1 onion, peeled and chopped
1/2oz (15g) sage leaves
2 garlic cloves
7oz (200g) risotto rice

I litre hot vegetable stock
Ifloz (30ml) olive oil salt & pepper
A pinch of nutmeg

◼ *Preparation*

1. Peel and deseed the butternut squash and cut into cubes. Fry with the onion in some of the olive oil, over a medium heat for six to eight minutes.
2. Chop three sprigs of sage, then add to the pan with the garlic and rice.
3. Add the chickpeas and a couple of ladles of stock and keep stirring until absorbed. Repeat until all stock is absorbed and the rice is tender – approximately twenty minutes. Season with salt and pepper.
4. Meanwhile, heat the rest of the olive oil in a small frying pan and add four sprigs of sage, cooking for twenty seconds, until crisp.
5. Serve the risotto, with the pinch of nutmeg and the fried sprigs of sage sprinkled on top.

Chicken pizzas – serves 2-4

Cute and scrumptious. These little chicken pizzas are great for those who need a protein boost. Don't forget to add a yummy side order to keep you filled up.

Ingredients

4 chicken breasts
I tube tomato puree
1/2 cup chopped peppers
1/2 cup onion
1/4 cup goat's cheese

◼ *Preparation*

1. Butterfly cut the chicken breasts and flatten them out.
2. Cover with tomato puree.
3. Sprinkle peppers and onions over the top.
4. Place on a baking tray in a pre-heated oven at 200°C for fifteen minutes.
5. Remove from the oven and sprinkle with goat's cheese.
6. Place them back in the oven for five minutes.
7. Serve with side dish of choice.

Brown rice and vegetable bake

A delicious vegetarian dish that will leave you feeling full and satisfied.

Ingredients

- 1 cup brown rice
- 2 onions, finely sliced
- 1 tbsp olive oil
- 10 Swiss chard leaves
- 5 eggs
- 1/2 teaspoon salt
- black pepper
- 3/4 cup freshly grated reduced-fat cheese
- 2 tomatoes, sliced

Preparation

1. Preheat oven to 180°C. Lightly oil a 10inch/25cm-round baking dish with a low-calorie oil spray.
2. Cook rice following packet directions.
3. Fry the onions in oil until soft and slightly caramelised. Remove white stalks from the chard and discard. Cook leaves on high in the microwave for two minutes. Squeeze out and moisture then chop.
4. Combine all of the ingredients except a handful of cheese and tomatoes. Spoon into the prepared dish and even out. Arrange the tomato slices on top and sprinkle with the remaining cheese.
5. Bake in the oven for about thirty-five to forty minutes or until firm in the middle and lightly browned.

Asparagus & Mushroom Quiche with Sweet Potato Crust

A scrummy quiche with a twist.

Ingredients

- 8 eggs, beaten
- 2 cups mushrooms, sautéed
- 1 bunch asparagus spears, sautéed
- 1/2 cup grape tomatoes
- 1/2 cup heirloom tomatoes
- Spiralized sweet potato (about 2-3 cups)
- salt and pepper

■ *Preparation*

1. Sauté the sweet potato in coconut oil, salt and pepper
2. Line a greased glass 9-inch pie dish with the sweet potatoes. Top with eggs, mushrooms, asparagus. Don't forget you can use as many or as few veggies as you like.
3. Cook at 180°C for twenty to twenty-fine minutes or until centre has set.

Fish parcels – serves 4

These fish parcels are quick to prepare and divine to eat. Adding different flavours to them is a great way of learning which foods you might like.

Ingredients

4 fish fillets of choice (salmon, cod, etc)
4 cloves of garlic, finely chopped
I medium red chili, finely chopped
7oz (200g) broccoli
7oz (200g) mange tout
4tbsp soy sauce

Side dish of choice
Vegetables
Rice noodles
Salad
Brown rice

■ *Preparation*

1. Heat the oven to 180°C. Lay each fish fillet onto a piece of tinfoil.
2. Spread with the garlic and chili. Lay the mange tout and broccoli over the fish and add the soy sauce to vegetables.
3. Wrap the tin foil around each individual fish parcel and ensure no gaps by keeping the foil tightly closed
4. Put the fish parcels into the oven for ten to fifteen minutes, check the fish is cooked to your taste before serving.
5. Serve with a side dish of brown rice, stir fried vegetables, salad or rice noodles.

Goa's cheese and asparagus frittata – serves 4

Goat's cheese is one of the healthiest cheeses you can consume and the perfect partner for asparagus.

Ingredients

    14oz (400g) asparagus tips
    1tbsp olive oil
    1 round of goat's cheese, crumbled
    6 large eggs
    Salad leaves of your choice

■ *Preparation*

1. Preheat the grill to medium-high. Cook the asparagus in a pan of simmering salted water, remove after five minutes when still tender and bright green. Put under a cold tap and cut into one centimentre pieces.
2. Lightly beat the eggs, adding the asparagus and chives. Season well.
3. Pour the egg mixture into the pan. Cook over a gentle heat for two minutes and then add the cheese, place under the grill for a few minutes or until lightly golden and the top is set.

Coconut chicken – serves 4

A great recipe for those who enjoy sweet food.

Ingredients

    11floz (300ml) coconut milk
    2tbsp tomato puree
    2tbsp ground almonds
    2tsp turmeric
    2tsp cumin
    4 chicken breast fillets, cut into small pieces
    2 onions, chopped
    2 cloves garlic, crushed
    2tbsp coconut oil

■ *Preparation*

1. Mix the coconut milk with the tomato puree, almonds, turmeric, cumin and one tablespoon of water. Add the chicken and coat well. Cover with cling film and refrigerate for at least one hour.
2. Cook the onions and garlic in teaspoon of coconut oil until soft.
3. Take the chicken from the marinade, add the onion to the pan, cover and cook for

two minutes over a low heat. Add the marinade and the remaining oil and cook for fifteen to twenty minutes.

4. Stir in fresh coriander and serve.

Favourite fishcakes – serves 2

Ingredients

1 rainbow trout
3 1/2oz (100g) smoked salmon
2 large sweet potatoes
1 small soft goat's cheese
2 cloves garlic, crushed
1 red chili diced
1 beaten egg
2oz (50g) gluten-free bread crumbs

Preparation

1. Wrap the trout in foil and place in oven for twenty-five minutes at 200°C.
2. Once it is cooked, leave to cool.
3. Peel and boil the sweet potatoes, then mash and leave to cool. Flake the trout into the mash, watching out for any sneaky bones. Cut the smoked salmon into small pieces and add to mash. Then add the garlic and chili.
4. Mix the ingredients together and leave in the fridge for no more than two hours.
5. When ready to eat, remove from fridge. Beat an egg in one bowl, and put breadcrumbs in another. Shape the fish mixture into cakes using your hands.
6. Place the fishcake into the bowl of beaten egg until covered, then into the bowl of breadcrumbs until completely covered. Repeat until all your mixture is used.
7. Bake the fishcakes in the oven for twenty-minutes to half an hour until golden brown. Serve with baby spinach or salad drizzled with balsamic vinegar and olive oil.

Cheese and bean quesadillas – serves 2-4

A satisfying and substantial Mexican dish which you can make from store cupboard ingredients.

Ingredients

4tbsp olive oil
2 small onions, chopped
4 cloves garlic, crushed

1 tsp chili powder
2 14oz (400g) tins kidney beans, rinsed and drained
8 medium tomatoes
4 wholemeal tortilla wraps
3oz (80g) Cheddar cheese
8 spring onions, thinly sliced
Salad leaves to garnish

■ *Preparation*

1. Heat olive oil in a pan and add the onion, cook until soft and brown. Add in the garlic and chili powder and then the beans and tomatoes and cook for four minutes until heated through.
2. Bake the tortillas for eight minutes in an oven at 200°C. Spoon the bean mixture onto the tortillas and then sprinkle over the cheese and spring onion, top this with another tortilla and press down to hold them firmly together with no gaps.
3. Bake for a further few minutes turning half way through.
4. Cut the quesadilla in half and serve with salad garnish.

Healthy cottage pie – serves 4

A twist on the traditional cottage pie which substitutes mince for turkey mince or Quorn. Both are great substitutes in this delicious family favourite.

Ingredients

1lb (500g) turkey mince or Quorn
4 sweet potatoes
2 sliced carrots
1 large onion
10 mushrooms
Wheat or gluten-free gravy mix
Coconut cooking oil
Dried mixed herbs

■ *Preparation*

1. Pre-heat the oven to 180°C for twenty minutes. Peel the sweet potatoes, chop and place in a pan of boiling water. Leave potatoes to boil for twenty minutes until soft.
2. Chop the onion, mushrooms and carrots. Heat a deep pan with one teaspoon of coconut oil. Add the onions and mushrooms, stir for two to three minutes until slightly golden. Add the turkey mince or Quorn to the pan and cook for around ten minutes until brown.
3. Add one teaspoon of mixed herbs and the carrots, then dissolve four heaped

tablespoons of gravy mix in 250ml of boiling water and add to the mince or Quorn.

4. Let it simmer, stirring occasionally, for approximately ten minutes.
5. Mash the sweet potatoes until smooth. Put the mince into an ovenproof dish then cover with the sweet potato and place in oven for around thirty minutes until the potatoes are crispy on the top.
6. Serve with cabbage or spring greens.

Chicken parmesan

Do you love breadcrumbs? Try this chicken dish but make your own. Pre-made breadcrumbs or those in processed food are an especially unhealthy choice as they are high in salt. Making your own will reduce this and taste better too.

Ingredients

1/2 cup grated parmesan cheese
1/2 cup wholewheat breadcrumbs
1 1/4lb thin chicken cutlets
1/4 cup plain non-fat Greek yogurt
1/4tsp dried oregano
1 lb tomatoes
1/4 cup red onion, finely chopped
1/4 cup fresh basil leaves, chopped
2tbsp extra virgin olive oil
1 clove garlic
1/2tsp crushed red pepper
8oz shredded fresh mozzarella

Preparation

1. Preheat oven to 200°C. Spray a pan with cooking spray. Mix Parmesan and crumbs together in a large dish.
2. In a medium bowl, toss the chicken with the yogurt, oregano, and 1/4 teaspoon of salt. Coat the cutlets in the crumb mixture, pressing to make sure all the crumbs stick, and place in the prepared pan. Sprinkle remaining crumbs on top of the cutlets; spray with cooking spray. Bake ten to fifteen minutes or until cooked through. While waiting make the salsa: mix the tomatoes, onion, basil, oil, garlic, red pepper, 1/4 teaspoon of salt, and 1/8 teaspoon of black pepper in a medium bowl. Place in the refrigerator for up to two hours.
3. Sprinkle mozzarella over tops of hot chicken and spoon tomato salsa mixture on top.

Grilled pork chops and melon salsa

Pork can become dry but adding a healthy sauce will make it so much tastier.

Ingredients

Salsa:
1 cup seedless watermelon, chopped
1 cup honeydew melon, chopped
3tbsps onion, finely chopped
1tbsp jalapeño pepper, finely chopped
1tbsp fresh coriander, chopped
1tbsp fresh lime juice

Pork chops:
2tsps rapeseed oil
1 1/2tsps chili powder
1/2tsps garlic powder
1/2tsps salt
1/4tsps freshly ground black pepper
4 boneless centre-cut pork chops, trimmed

■ *Preparation*

1.   1. Combine the ingredients for the salsa and set aside.
2.   Heat a griddle pan over medium-high heat. Combine oil, chilli and garlic powder, salt and pepper in a bowl and rub this over both sides of the pork chops. Spray pan with oil.
3.   Add chops to pan and cook four minutes on each side. Serve with salsa and maybe a salad too.

Grilled chicken with peaches

A fruit with chicken? Its ingenious and this dish is one I really suggest you try. It really is beautiful.

Ingredients

4 boneless skinless chicken breasts
1/2 cup fresh basil leaves, chopped
4 peaches, halved with stone removed

Marinade
1/2 cup peach preserve
1/2 cup olive oil
1/4 cup apple cider vinegar
3tbsp lemon juice

2tbsp course grain Dijon mustard
1 garlic clove, crushed
1/2tsp salt
1/4tsp pepper

▪ *Preparation*

1. Rinse the chicken and set aside.
2. Lightly spray peaches with olive oil and set aside.
3. Combine marinade ingredients and whisk well. Set half a cup aside for basting.
4. Add chicken to remaining marinad, cover with cling film and marinate for at least two hours.
5. When ready, heat grill to medium to high.
6. Add chicken and peaches to grill and discard the marinade.
7. Grill for around fifteen minutes turning the chicken once halfway through.
8. Serve with a salad and whole grain rice.

Mini spinach cannelloni

Cannelloni can be healthy if you do not add copious amounts of salt and cheese, if you use cheese just limit the amounts – a serving of cheese is 20g, about the size of a matchbox, and you should have no more than three servings a day – or swap to a low fat cheese. These mini cannelloni are perfect for maintaining portion control.

Ingredients

9 sheets of lasagne, cooked
10oz packet frozen chopped spinach, thawed and completely drained
15oz fat free ricotta
1/2 cup grated Parmesan cheese
1 egg
1/2tsp minced garlic
1/2tsp dried Italian seasoning
salt and fresh pepper
1 chicken breast, cooked and diced
32oz tomato pasta sauce
9 tbsp low-fat mozzarella, shredded

▪ *Preparation*

1. Preheat oven to 180°C. Make sure you drain the spinach well.
2. Combine spinach, ricotta, Parmesan cheese, egg, garlic, Italian seasoning, chicken, and salt and pepper in a medium bowl.
3. Pour about one cup of tomato sauce on the bottom of a 9 x 13 baking dish.4.

Place a piece of wax paper on your worktop and lay out the sheets of lasagne. Make sure they are dry by patting them lightly with a paper towel.

4.   Take a third of a cup of ricotta mixture and spread evenly over a sheet of lasagne. Roll carefully and place seam side down onto the baking dish. Repeat with remaining sheets.

5.   Ladle the remaining tomato sauce over the cannelloni and top each one with one tablespoon of mozzarella. Cover the baking dish tightly with tin foil and bake for twenty to thirty minutes, or until the cheese melts.

Healthy sweet and sour chicken

Instead of a readymade sweet and sour sauce from a jar, try creating your own with this recipe. It's much healthier and tastier.

Ingredients

2 skinless boneless chicken breasts
I tbsp olive oil

Sauce:
1/4 cup rice wine vinegar
3tbsps honey
2tbsps tomato paste
I tsp fresh grated ginger
2 garlic cloves, minced
I tsp garlic
1/2 orange, squeezed
Salt and pepper to taste

■   *Preparation*

1.   Cut chicken breast into cubes and season with salt and pepper.

2.   Griddle the chicken breasts in a preheated pan rubbed with the olive oil – about five to ten minutes. Set aside.

3.   Make sauce, by adding all ingredients into a small saucepan and bringing to the boil, then reduce to a simmer until sauce thickens.

4.   Toss the chicken in the sauce until it is well–coated. Serve with rice or quinoa topped with steamed veggies, grated raw carrot and the chicken.

Turkey tangine

Try this gorgeous tangine and remember that turkey is a good sauce of protein.

Ingredients

1lb (450g) diced turkey
2tbsp seasoned flour
1tbsp olive oil
1 onion, diced
3 garlic cloves, crushed
1tsp ground coriander
1tsp ground cinnamon
3 1/2oz (100g) mushrooms, sliced
14oz (400g) tin chickpeas, drained
14oz (400g) tin chopped tomatoes
1pint (450ml) low-salt turkey or chicken stock
2 1/2oz (75g) dried apricots
1tbsp fresh coriander, chopped

For the Couscous
8oz (225g) cous cous
1tsp ground cinnamon
1tbsp toasted flaked almonds
1tbsp fresh coriander, chopped

■ *Preparation*

1. Toss the turkey in the seasoned flour. Heat the oil in a large pan and gently sauté the onion, garlic and spices for five minutes. Add the turkey and continue to cook, stirring for around three minutes.
2. Add the flour and mushrooms and cook for a further two minutes. Then stir in the drained chickpeas, canned tomatoes with their juice and the stock. Bring to the boil, cover with a lid then reduce heat and simmer for ten minutes.
3. Add the apricots to the chicken and cook for a further ten to fifteen minutes or until the turkey is tender.
4. While waiting, cover the couscous with 450ml (1 pint) of boiling water. Leave for ten to fifteen minutes, stirring occasionally or until the water has been absorbed. Stir occasionally to separate the grains. Stir in the ground cinnamon and chopped coriander.
5. To serve spoon the chicken on top of the couscous, sprinkle with the toasted flaked almonds and chopped coriander.

I hope these recipes gave you some insight into what healthy eating can be. It does not mean eating nothing and does not restrict the range of foods you can eat, it means swapping foods and cutting out processed foods and salt. I want you to enjoy your meals and not dread cooking them. And I hope it gave you some inspiration. Next on our list is side dishes.

SIDE DISHES

Sometimes when planning meals it can be hard to keep thinking up a variety of side dishes. Steamed vegetables and salads can get a bit boring after a while and obviously chips and fried foods are off the menu. Here are some suggestions to make them more tempting and to help you ring the changes. They might even inspire you to create your own.

Baked courgettes

Courgettes are cheap and easy to prepare. Once you have tried and tested this, I think you will use this frequently as it is quick to make. It is so delicious you could serve it for a summer lunch with a salad.

Ingredients

> Olive oil for greasing
> 2 medium-sized courgettes
> I onion
> 2 eggs
> Pinch nutmeg
> Ground pepper
> 1/2 cup low-fat grated cheese

■ *Preparation*

1. Preheat the oven to 200°C.
2. Trim the courgettes but do not peel. Grate them and the peeled onion and add to the lightly beaten eggs. Season with nutmeg and pepper. Spoon into a lightly greased ovenproof dish and sprinkle with cheese.
3. Bake in the oven for fifteen minutes until the cheese is melted and golden.

Garlic roasted cabbage

Create a different taste to cabbage with this great little method.

Ingredients

> I big green cabbage, chopped into thick slices
> 3tbsp extra-virgin olive oil
> 5 large garlic cloves, chopped
> Sea salt and freshly ground black pepper to taste

■ *Preparation*

1. Preheat your oven to 180°C.
2. Brush both sides of each cabbage slice with olive oil.
3. Spread the garlic evenly on each side of the cabbage slices, and season with salt and pepper.
4. Roast in the oven for twenty minutes, turn the slices and continue to roast until crispy

Sweet potato wedges

Simple and sweet and the perfect substitute for chips. Don't forget all the nutrients contained in these lovely little nuggets.

Ingredients

4 sweet potatoes, cooked through and cut into slices
Olive oil
2-3tsp Dijon mustard
Pepper

■ *Preparation*

1. Parboil the sweet potatoes for around ten minutes.
2. Drain the potatoes and let them dry. Rub with the mustard.
3. Grill or bake for around ten minutes or until golden brown and season with pepper to taste.

Chilli side

We think of chilli as a main course but this vegetable side dish is a delicious accompaniment to a main meal. It's full of protein and you could even refrigerate it for lunch the next day .

Ingredients

I onion, chopped
Itbsp olive oil 14oz (400g) tin black beans
14oz (400g) tin red kidney beans
1/2 cup red lentils
14oz (400g) tin chopped tomatoes
Itbsp tomato paste
I courgette, grated
I carrot, grated
¾ cup vegetable or chicken stock (low sodium)
1/2tsp ground cumin

1/2tsp smoked paprika
1/2tsp chilli flakes

■ *Preparation*

1. Gently fry the onion and garlic in the oil until soft. Add all the other ingredients to the pot and stir well to combine. Bring to a simmer, then cook for around twenty minutes, until the lentils are soft and mushy and the liquid has evaporated.
2. Serve with your dish of choice.

Low-fat coleslaw

A crunchy nutritious delight you can enjoy guilt-free.

Ingredients

1lb (about 500g) shredded cabbage
4 spring onions, sliced
2 large carrots, peeled and grated
2 stalks celery, sliced
1/2 cup reduced-fat mayonnaise
1/2 cup low-fat plain yogurt
2tbsps white vinegar
4tsps honey

■ *Preparation*

1. Mix the cabbage, spring onions, carrots and celery together in a large bowl.
2. Combine the mayonnaise, yogurt, vinegar and honey in a medium bowl. Combine with the cabbage mixture. Season with freshly ground black pepper.

Crunchy apple dip

Ingredients

2 apples, sliced thinly
1tbsp raw honey
1tbsp hemp seeds
2tsps all natural almond butter
Dash of cinnamon

■ *Preparation*

1. Combine all the ingredients and serve with the sliced apples.

DESSERTS

Since we are creatures of habit, it's inevitable we will get cravings for sweet things every now and then. With careful planning you should be able to have your (low-fat) cake – and eat it too.

Avocado chocolate mousse

Who knew puddings could be healthy and scrummy. This exquisite little dessert is like a little bowl of heaven. Definitely one to try.

Ingredients
- I ripe avocado
- 1/4 cup cocoa powder
- 1/4 cup raw agave nectar
- 1/4 cup almond milk
- I tsp vanilla

■ *Preparation*
1. Remove the skin and stone from the avocado and slice into chunks.
2. Place into a food processor with the rest of the ingredients and process until smooth. Ensure all ingredients are mixed in well.
3. Place into serving dishes and serve.

Apple crisp

Using one of your five-a-day to enjoy a treat.

Ingredients
- 4 cups apples, peeled and thinly sliced
- 1/4 cup coconut milk
- 2tsp lemon juice
- I tsp cinnamon

Crumble topping
- 1/4 cup coconut flour
- 1/4 cup almond flour
- 4tsp chopped nuts
- I tsp coconut oil
- I tsp salt

■ *Preparation*

1. Preheat oven to 190°C.
2. Mix together the apples, lemon juice, coconut milk and cinnamon.
3. Using your hands, combine all the crumble ingredients in a separate bowl – add more coconut oil if mixture is a little dry.
4. Grease a baking dish.
5. Pour the apple mixture into the dish and evenly spread the crumble topping over the apples.
6. Bake for approximately twenty-five minutes, ensuring the apples are tender and then serve while warm.

Chocolate chia cookies

If you are a chocolate lover or a biscuit lover – or both, then this recipe is most definitely for you.

Ingredients

    1 cup almonds
    1 cup hazelnuts
    1 cup quinoa
    1/3 cup pure maple syrup
    1/4 cup dates
    3tsp raw cacao powder
    2tsp coconut oil
    2tsp chia seed
    1 cup water

■ *Preparation*

1. Blend the nuts in a food processor to make a flour. Add the rest of the ingredients until a sticky dough is formed.
2. Scoop a tablespoon of the mixture into your hand and roll into a ball, then flatten it. Place onto a baking tray. Repeat for the rest of the mixture.
3. Put into the oven and bake at 180°C until browned and firm, around ten to fifteen minutes.

Frozen blueberry pineapple Greek yogurt bark

A must-try that tastes as good as it looks.

Ingredients

    2 cups plain Greek yogurt
    1/4 cup honey

1 tsp vanilla extract
2 cups fresh blueberries, washed and cleaned
1/2 cup pineapple chunks
You could also use flavoured yogurt and omit the honey

Preparation

1. Line a 9 x 13 cake tin with parchment or wax paper.
2. Mix together yogurt, vanilla and honey.
3. Add blueberries and pineapple.
4. Stir until the fruit is evenly coated.
5. Spread out evenly on parchment lined pan.
6. Freeze overnight.

Healthy ice cream

This is a healthy version of ice cream with only four ingredients. This would also make a great dessert to serve up after dinner.

Ingredients

2 bananas, cut into one inch slices (frozen)
1/2 cup frozen strawberries, sliced
2 tbsp almond milk
1/2 tsp vanilla

You can use any frozen fruit to make this, so have fun playing with different flavours.

Preparation

1. Place banana slices on a plate, separating each slice. Place slices in freezer for at least two hours – overnight is best.
2. Remove strawberries and bananas from freezer and blend in a food processor until they are the consistency of soft-serve ice cream.
3. Add the almond milk and vanilla until you reach the desired texture and blend until smooth.
4. Transfer ice cream to a freezer container and freeze until solid.
5. Serve with fresh strawberries.

TREATS

I love this little section full of ideas so good you won't want to eat them. I hope you enjoy them.

Yogurt parfait

Ingredients

6oz plain or low-fat yogurt
1/2 cup unsweetened frozen berries
1/2 cup of granola (see recipe on page 124)
2tbsp flaked almonds

Preparation

1. Layer the ingredients into pretty glasses and serve

Raspberry ice lollies – Serves 4

Ingredients

2 1/2oz (75g) raspberry jelly (about half a packet)
8 1/2floz (250ml) boiling water
3 1/2oz (100g) fresh raspberries
5floz (150g) vanilla drinking yogurt

Preparation

1. Dissolve the raspberry jelly in a bowl with boiling water, stirring well, then transfer to the fridge for about two hours to set.
2. Push the raspberries through a sieve, discarding the leftover seeds. Combine the raspberry juice and yogurt in a blender. Add the jelly, pulse for a minute or two till well combined – the mixture does not need to be completely smooth.
3. Pour the mixture into lolly moulds or ice cube trays. Insert lolly sticks, then cover with cling film.
4. Freeze for at least nine hours or overnight.

Apple cinnamon yogurt pancakes – Serves 4 (eight pancakes)

Love pancakes and don't want to miss out? This healthy, tasty version is sure to take away sweet cravings.

Ingredients

1 egg
1 cup plain non-fat yogurt

1tbsp low-calorie spray oil
1 cup flour
1tsp baking powder
1/2tsp baking soda
1tsp cinnamon
Pinch salt
3 cups apple, peeled and sliced
2tbsp honey or maple syrup

▪ *Preparation*

1. Combine the egg, yogurt, oil and a tablespoon of the honey or maple syrup in a blender until smooth (or mix with a whisk or fork).
2. Sift together the flour, baking soda, baking powder, cinnamon and salt.
3. Add to the yogurt mixture and blend. Spray a frying pan with cooking oil spray and heat over a medium heat.
4. Ladle the mixture into the pan to make eight small pancakes – you might find it easier to do this in batches.
5. Cook until bubbles appear (about one to two minutes) and then flip.
6. Divide the pancakes onto four plates and top with the sliced apple and a drizzle of the remaining honey or maple syrup.

Flower ice lollies

This idea is fantastic. The lollies are so tasty and appealing. Your family and friends will definitely be impressed and wanting the recipe.

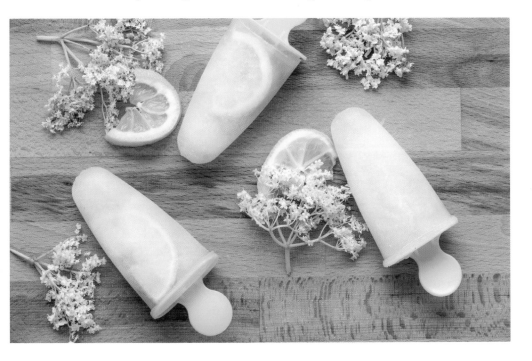

Ingredients

> 1 pint (455ml) cold water
> 1floz (30ml) orange blossom water
> 1tsp lemon juice
> Handful of organic edible flower petals available from selected supermarkets
>   and online.

■ *Preparation*

1.   Have the ice lolly moulds handy and make sure you have room in your freezer.
2.   Combine the water, orange blossom water and lemon juice. Sweeten to taste.
3.   Pour mixture into the moulds. Freeze without sticks or petals for about an hour.
4.   Remove from freezer and add the flower petals. You can push them into the
     moulds with the help of a long, skinny spoon or pop stick. Make sure the flowers
     are scattered throughout the lollies.
5.   Add the sticks and freeze for two to three hours until solid.

Edible flowers can be used to brighten up other dishes too and also look great in
ice cubes. Try livening up your food with these dainty additions.

SNACKS

Snacks don't have to be boring. You can see your healthy eating plan as a chance
to create new snack ideas and make them fun. Fruit kebabs are a great way
to enjoy a variety of fruits and fruit salad is perfect for trying out exotic new
flavours. We make healthy eating creative and fun for children so why not for
adults too.

Let us look at this list of snacks and see if you can be tempted by some new
ideas;

Asparagus wrapped in ham

Boiled eggs

Cereal – add fruit, nuts, seeds and yogurt

Crisps – spiced pear, beet, baked crisps, kale (available in health food shops
or make your own)

Dried fruit – prunes, apricots, figs are handy for a snack on the go

Fresh fruit – make fruit salads, fruit kebabs, yogurts, smoothies, ice lollies
and even jelly

Mushrooms stuffed with low-fat cream cheese

Nuts – pistachios, almond, walnuts, pecans

Oatcakes – spread with nut butter and the fruit of choice. Or low-fat cream cheese and cucumber. Offer a variety of toppings in separate bowls and let family or guests help themselves. Delicious!

Pancakes – add fruit or natural syrup or honey for flavour

Peanut butter on apples, strawberries on bagels, banana on toast, tomatoes stuffed with low-fat cream cheese

Popcorn (unsalted and without butter)

Rice cakes – see oatcakes

Seed mix – pumpkin seeds, flax, sunflower seeds

Vegetables – carrots, celery, asparagus are another great on-the-go snack

Yogurt – natural, organic, frozen

So now you have looked at the various foods. Let us now look at the health properties of fruit and vegetables. In the next chapter I have listed alphabetically all the fruits and vegetables I think you'll enjoy.

CHAPTER 8

A-Z OF FOODS AND THEIR BENEFITS AND CALORIE COUNTERS

'If you do not recognise an ingredient, your body won't either.'

So I have spoken about superfoods, calories, sugar and salt. I have given you some of my favourite recipes but I keep talking about fruits and veggies and spices, so this chapter is dedicated to explaining why these foods are good for us and a table at the end gives their calorie contents.

Apples: According to studies, quercetin, an antioxidant found in apples, helps reduce bad cholesterol oxidation. Apples are rich in a soluble fibre called pectin. There are studies which suggest that this may be able to help to reduce levels of toxic heavy metals within the body. Apples have also shown to fill us up so they make great snacks for weight-loss.

Apricots: Apricots contain high beta-carotene which makes them an important heart health food; the beta-carotene helps protect our cholesterol from oxidation, which may in turn help to prevent heart disease. Apricots contain vitamin B2, potassium, and magnesium. They also contain iron and copper, which are extremely important for keeping our blood healthy and helping to prevent us from getting an iron deficiency.

Asparagus: Asparagus is a good source of folic acid which is important for pregnant women. It is also full of antioxidants, which as we know helps with cell-damaging free radicals, making it a great anti-aging vegetable. Asparagus is a great source of fibre, vitamins A, C, E and K, as well as chromium, a mineral that may assist insulin to carry glucose from the bloodstream into our cells. With all these healthy properties, it's not surprising that asparagus has been dubbed a superfood.

Aubergine: Aubergines are low in calories and sodium and contain a phytochemical called monoterpene that may help prevent cancer cell growth. Studies have shown it helps with controlling high blood pressure too.

Avocado: As I discussed earlier this is another superfood. Avocados are full of flavour and are great to eat if you're craving something fatty and sweet. They have high potassium levels so they help to keep our blood pressure low. They also contain mono-unsaturated fats that help to lower blood pressure.

Bananas: Bananas are a good source of B vitamins, which may help to treat insomnia, mood swings and irritability. They also contain vitamin C, as well as magnesium and potassium, which make them great energy-boosting foods. Due to their fibre content they are excellent aids to digestion. They are high in natural sugars, so rather than reaching for sweet junk foods, have a banana to satisfy sweet cravings. Bananas are a good base for smoothies.

Beets: Numerous studies have shown that beets can help oxygenate blood and enhance exercise performance. Beets are a good source of phytonutrients antioxidants and folic acid, and also contain vitamins A and C, choline, iodine, manganese, organic sodium, potassium and fibre.

Bell peppers: All peppers have health benefits but the red bell pepper in particular is health-giving as it contains beta-carotene. It is also rich in vitamin C, which helps to repair our bodies and improve oral hygiene, and vitamin A, which helps keep our eyes and skin healthy. Antioxidants in peppers help to protect against heart disease and some cancers.

Blackberries: These are one of the highest sources of antioxidants, which is great for our skin, as well as being an excellent source of vitamin C, fibre, iron, calcium, manganese and potassium. They are very low in calories so make great snacks for dieters.

Blueberries: These contain pectin, vitamin C, potassium, flavonoids and important amounts of tannins, which can kill bacteria and fight off infections. Consuming these little berries is associated with a decreased risk of type-2 diabetes.

Blackcurrants: A recent study completed by Dundee University showed that these contained sixty-eight times more antioxidants than other berries, and have been shown to improve blood flow around our body. They contain antioxidants called anthocyanins, which give them their distinctive dark purple colour. The darker the blackcurrant, the more anthocyanins it contains and the more beneficial it is for you. Blackcurrants are especially rich in vitamin C – containing more than three times as much as an orange. They are perfect for smoothies and fruit salads and make excellent ice cream.

Broccoli: Broccoli is a vegetable known to benefit the liver and promote natural detoxification. As mentioned before broccoli is a superfood because of its many health benefits.

Cabbage: Contains sulphur, which purifies our blood, and is one of very few vegetables that contains vitamin E which keeps the hair and skin healthy. It comes in various colours such as purple, white and green and is worth adding to your plate each week due to its low calorie count.

Cantaloupes: These sweet and tasty melons are very low in calories and packed full of nutrition. They have high levels of beta-carotene, folic acid, potassium, vitamin C, and fibre as well as a vast amount of the vitamin B compound – unlike most other fruits and vegetables. Many people forget about these little beauties.

Carrots: Widely available and a great source of vitamins A, B, and C. They are rich in beta-carotene and carotenoids and studies suggest they can help prevent cardiac disease. They also contain iron, calcium, potassium and natural sodium. My parents used to say if you eat your carrots you will be able to see in the dark. They are the dieter's friend as they help with weight-loss and are low in calories.

Celery: A great low-calorie food. The high levels of silicon in celery can help to strengthen joints, bones, arteries and connective tissues. It is high in minerals so including this veggie as part of a healthy diet may help promote healthy blood pressure and cholesterol. Studies have shown that it can help reduce migraines too.

Cherries: Contains iron and helps to strengthen blood. Cherries contain vitamins A and C as well as biotin and potassium. Cherries can help improve sleep and are great for weight-loss due to their low calorie count.

Cranberries: Cranberries are high in antioxidants so they are great for our skin and they also contain proanthocyanidins, which are known to support overall health. The other nutrients they contain could protect against tooth cavities and studies have shown it can help with urinary tract infections and inflammatory diseases. Cranberries are a diuretic so can help to flush excess water and toxins from the body.

Cucumbers: Cucumber is my favourite food. They contain potassium, which can help lower cholesterol and their high water content makes them perfect for juicing or as a low calorie snack to keep us hydrated. Cucumbers are good for digestive problems and thin slices are very soothing for tired eyes.

Dandelion: Very high in vitamin K, which is important for blood and bone health. Dandelion is a diuretic, and is very beneficial for the kidneys.

Dates: Rich in vitamins, minerals and fibre and high in calcium, potassium and iron. Great if you are looking to gain weight and for our digestive system.

Fennel: Fennel contains high levels of vitamin C, as well as folic acid, potassium and fibre. It is not spoken about much, but it is a low-calorie vegetable, great antioxidant, an anti-inflammatory food and its great advantage is that it is easy to juice!

Grapefruits: High in vitamin C. Quite a tangy taste but great for a juice but not daily. It can help aid weight-loss and also bowel movement. Grapefruits are great for boosting your immune system.

Grapes: Grapes contain vitamins A, B, C and folic acid, and contain many important minerals like potassium, calcium, iron, phosphorus, magnesium and selenium. The flavonoids found in grapes have antioxidant properties that can lessen the damage caused by free radicals, which help in the anti-aging process. They are perfect for healthy snacking.

Jalapeno: This is actually a form of fruit, believe it or not, but is used as a vegetable. It can help with sinusitis but is also great for weight-loss as it is an appetite suppressant.

Kale: We have spoken about kale earlier and its low-calorie, nutrition-rich advantages. Kale is a major player in our leafy green family.

Kiwi fruit: I love this fruit but many people are put off it because of its brown furry skin. Kiwis are excellent source of vitamin C. Vitamin C helps to keep teeth and gums healthy. Eating kiwi fruits can boost our immune system and studies have shown that they boost digestion and are high in fibre.

Leeks: Leeks are rich in antioxidants and phytonutrients. They are great for detoxing the body and studies have suggested they can assist with anaemia.

Lemons: This fruit is high in vitamin C. Lemons and limes contain limonene, which may help to prevent breast cancer as well as a natural anti-emetic and properties to aid digestion. Lemon is great for detoxing the body and aiding weight-loss as well as boosting our immunity.

Limes: These contain vitamin C, vitamin B6, folic acid, potassium, flavonoids and many other phytonutrients. This citrus fruit is great for detoxing our body and can also help with boosting immunity and increasing energy.

Mangos: This exotic fruit is an excellent source of vitamins A and C, which helps to maintain a strong immune system. Mangos contain a great deal of flavonoids like beta-carotene, alpha-carotene and beta-cryptoxanthin. According to some studies, mango also alkalises the body.

Melons: These are great for a snack when you're craving sweetness while dieting.

Onions: Onions contain a naturally occurring chemical which has been found to promote bone health. They contain high levels of quercetin, an antioxidant that lessens free radical damage. Red onions can also help to lower blood sugar levels. Phytochemicals within onions improve vitamin C levels within the body and boost our immunity. It is also a natural anti-inflammatory and helps heal infections and has been traditionally used as a complementary medicine.

Oranges: Excellent sources of vitamin C. They keep us hydrated and are excellent for juicing. Its high fibre content aids digestion and apparently the skin is also good for curing hangovers. It is good for our skin, fights the common cold and eases allergies.

Papayas: Can promote healthy digestion and regular bowel movements with their potent enzymes. They are high in vitamins A, C, and potassium, which means they can help with our eyesight. Like other fruits they are low in calories so aid weight-loss.

Parsnips: Good source of vitamins C and E, helps maintain healthy blood pressure and contains fibre which improves our bowel health.

Passionfruit: This tropical fruit is full of vitamins and phytonutrients. Health benefits are increased bone mineral density and good blood circulation. They are great for the skin and hair and can apparently help beat insomnia.

Peaches: Great source of vitamin A and potassium. Good for our skin and heart and low in calories, studies have shown peaches assist with liver and kidney function. Peaches are delicious but be mindful if buying tinned ones as the syrup is high in sugar.

Pears: A diuretic fruit that is rich in fibre and low in sodium. Great for digestive health and as an energy booster. I am partial to low-sugar poached pears as a dessert.

Pineapples: This fruit is beneficial for our immune system and digestive system as it is high in vitamins A and C. Pineapple contains bromelain which has protein-digesting properties and promotes natural detoxification.

Plums: These are rich in antioxidants and help with the anti-ageing process. They also help metabolic processes and ease constipation.

Pomegranate: Rich in tannins and flavonoids. Pomegranates are originally from the Middle East and are supposedly effective against heart disease and high blood pressures. Juice made from this fruit allegedly contains more antioxidants than red wine, green tea or blueberries.

Radishes: Great for the digestive system and very detoxifying. A great source of potassium and iron. Perfect on a salad.

Raspberries: Very high in antioxidants and a super immune booster, they contain potassium, niacin, iron and vitamin C.

Romaine lettuce: Romaine is rich in minerals and a great source of iron, especially for vegetarians. Low in calories but high in vitamins and calcium.

Spring onions: Great for boosting heart and eyesight, according to studies, and they are a flavoursome addition to salads.

Spinach: Rich in vitamin and minerals – Popeye was certainly right to consume this as studies show that it keeps our bones healthy, regulates blood pressure, helps with digestive system and boosts our immunity.

Strawberries: High in antioxidants and fabulous for our skin. An excellent source of vitamin C and great for weight-loss since they are mostly water.

Sugar-snap peas: A great source of riboflavin, vitamin B6, pantothenic acid, magnesium, phosphorus and potassium. They are also full of fibre so aid the digestive system and we can load our plate with these as they are low in calories.

Sweet potatoes: I love sweet potato. It's a superfood and lives up to its name with all its health properties and advantages.

Tomatoes: These contain vitamin C, as well as antioxidants that may prevent cancer, such as lycopene. Lycopene promotes overall mental and physical health. Tomatoes keep skin looking healthy, promote sound sleep and help control weight-loss. Stock up on lots of these as snacks.

Tangerines, mandarins, satsumas and clementines: Great little fruits that fill you up and aid digestion. All are high in vitamin C and great for our skin and also our hearts, as studies have shown. These are also really cheap and you get lots for your money.

Ugli: This fruit is originally from Jamaica and has great healthy benefits such as promoting oral hygiene and boosting immunity. It's higher in fibre than other fruits so it is great for the digestive system.

Knowing the benefits of fruits and veggies is important since this makes us more aware of why we should eat them. Next are herbs and spices, you may be thinking spices are just added to food for flavour, but what you may be unaware of is the health properties that come with them too. If you are told to cut back on salt, oil and other flavourings then spices are the ideal way to literally 'spice things up'. Let us have a look at some spices that may help you in more ways than one;

Basil: Bail is a soothing digestive, antibacterial, antidepressant and anti-inflammatory herb. Basil is a good source of magnesium, which assists our cardiovascular health by promoting healthy blood flow around our body.

Chinese five spice powder: a compound of five different spices all with great benefits. These are cloves, which are rich in vitamins and minerals; cinnamon which is a powerful antioxidant; Sichuan peppercorns, known for being rich in essential oils and antioxidants; star anise, which has antioxidant functions from vitamins A and C, plus B-complex vitamins, and finally fennel, an antioxidant rich in minerals, and known for easing the stomach and promoting smoother digestion. So what better way to add extra flavour and benefit our bodies.

Coriander: Coriander is known to be rich in antioxidants and dietary fibre, which can help to lower bad cholesterol and raise our good cholesterol levels. It's full of good things including folic acid, riboflavin, niacin, vitamin A, beta carotene, vitamin C and vitamin K. Preliminary investigation in mice suggests that a phytonutrient found in coriander, may be useful in managing Alzheimer's disease and improving memory. Studies in humans back this up with the benefit believed to come from coriander's vitamin K content.

Cinnamon: Known to help beat cravings, this spice may also reduce inflammation, have antioxidant effects and fight bacteria. It has already been shown to help keep blood sugar in check too. And it's delicious.

Dill: Dill is actually a herb from the celery family. It is packed with compounds called monoterpenes, flavonoids, minerals and certain amino acids, which have many medicinal properties. Health benefits are that it apparently soothes our digestive system, it can reduce insomnia, and supports healthy menstruation. Dill is a good source of vitamin A so not only are you adding a tangy slightly aniseedy taste to your meals, you are also consuming nutrients.

Garlic: I am a massive fan of garlic because you can add it to almost any meal to make it taste delicious. People sometimes avoid it because it can linger on the breath but it is widely used around the world and with good reason. Garlic is known to be an antimicrobial, an antibiotic, a diuretic and an antihistamine and it apparently lowers blood cholesterol levels and blood sugar levels. Garlic is known to have good sources of vitamins C and B6, manganese and selenium, so not only is it good as a vampire repellent it is good for keeping nasty diseases away too.

Ginger: Ginger is known to support healthy digestion and to cleanse in the body. Studies have shown it can help as an anti-emetic and an anti-inflammatory. Ginger has apparently been use in medicine for centuries and is used widely in Asian cuisine. Ideal for sweet and savoury dishes.

Jalapenos: Love or hate them they certainly are beneficial to us. Jalapenos contain capsaicin, which helps to fight migraines and nasty headaches. Eating them is also believed to help with nasal congestion and sinus infections. They can support our metabolism and can aid efficient fat burning too.

Mint: Mint is a great herb and there also many varieties, though they all support smooth digestion, as well as indigestion and inflammation. The scent of mint can help to stimulate our saliva glands to secrete digestive enzymes which improve our digestion. It is rich in plant-based omega-3 fats which are an important nutrient for healthy hair, skin, and nails, so all you ladies can add this herb into your diets for lovely locks and smooth skin.

Tarragon: A herb from the sunflower family which is used in dishes across the Mediterranean. Health benefits include helping to lower our blood glucose levels and it is a great source of vitamins C and A. Tarragon also contains calcium, manganese, iron, magnesium, copper, potassium and zinc. Tarragon has quite an intense liquorice flavour and is a perfect match for chicken.

Parsley: One of the most common herbs, you have probably come across it already as it used in all kinds of recipes and as a garnish too. Parsley does not just make our food taste nice it also contains one of the highest sources of vitamin C. It is believed to have diuretic properties, which means it helps the body to get rid of excess water. Rich in folic acid, it promotes heart health. Parsley is part of the celery family and its name comes from the Greek for 'rock celery'.

I find it amazing and fascinating to think of all these foods, herbs and spices and their advantages to our health. Some have been used for centuries as medicines so we are not the first to realise the benefits. Just think if they have all the properties medical studies have shown them to have, how healthy this world could be if we all consumed them regularly.

Throughout this book we have looked at our nutritional needs, calories, the foods to eat and those to avoid, so let us take a look at some of the calories in preparation for your shopping list. If you work out your calorie intake based on these figures, you may get an insight into why you put weight on.

As mentioned before, keeping track of your calorie intake is important as is known the calorific value of certain food. This is particularly useful if you choose to keep a record, but it will also show you the calories you consume now compared to the lower calories that you could consume and this will give you the motivation to succeed.

Food	Serving size/portion	Calorie
Orange fruit juice	5 floz (140ml)	50
Apple	3 1/2oz (100g)	47
Banana	3 1/2oz (100g)	95
Strawberry	1 (1/2oz/12g)	3

Food	Serving size/portion	Calorie
Orange	4oz (120g)	44
Blueberries	1tbsp	11
Blackberries	1	1
Pears	1 (6oz/170g)	90
Grapes (seedless)	1	1
Cucumber	1 inch (2oz/60g)	6
Lettuce	3 1/2oz (100g)	14
Tomatoes	1 (1/2oz/15g)	2
Celery	1 stick (1oz/30g)	2
Onion	1 slice (3/4oz/20g)	7
Carrot	3 1/2oz (100g)	35
Cauliflower	3 1/2oz (100g)	28
Broccoli	3 1/2oz (100g)	24
Peas	1tbsp (1oz/30g)	23
Asparagus	3 1/2oz (100g)	26
Chicken breast – without skin	3 1/2oz (100g)	148
Roasted Chicken	4 slices (1 1/2oz/40g)	280
Beef mince – without oil	3 1/2oz (100g)	183
Beef rump steak – grilled	3 1/2oz (100g)	177
Beef sirloin steak	3 1/2oz (100g)	176
Beef stewing steak	3oz (90g)	166
Grilled lamb steaks	2 1/2oz (70g)	138
Pork loin steaks	4oz (120g)	229
Sweet potato – baked	3 1/2oz (100g)	115
Sweet potato – steamed	3 1/2oz (100g)	84
Sweet potato fries	3 1/2oz (100g)	196
Potato – baked	3 1/2oz (100g)	136
Potato – mashed with butter	1 forkful – (1oz/30g)	31
New potatoes – in their skins and boiled in unsalted water	3 1/2oz (100g)	66
Brown organic rice	3 1/2oz (100g)	357

Food	Serving size/portion	Calorie
Egg fresh noodles	3 1/2oz (100g)	145
Long grain rice	3 1/2oz (100g)	136
Steamed salmon	3 1/2oz (100g)	194
Grilled salmon	3 1/2oz (100g)	215
Baked cod	1 3/4oz (50g)	48
Fish pie	9oz (250g)	297
Steamed cod	1 3/4oz (50g)	48
Fishcakes in batter	3 1/2oz (100g)	154
Poached cod	1 3/4oz (50g)	47
Grilled haddock	1 3/4oz (50g)	52
Tuna in brine	1 3/4oz (45g)	44
Tuna jacket potato with low-fat mayonnaise		370
Brown bread	3 1/2oz (100g)	252
Granary bread	3 1/2oz (100g)	235

It's a lot of information to take in, isn't it? However, this means that you now know the importance of eating fruit and veggies, and hopefully you have learnt something new with all the facts and information. I want to start you on your new lifestyle with so much inspiration that you feel really motivated to follow through on weight-loss plan and achieve your gaols. We will now put all this information together to create your plan.

CHAPTER 9
PUTTING THIS ALL TOGETHER

'A journey of a thousand miles starts with a single step.'

Lao Tzu

So after the chapters we have read we need to work out how to put all this information together. We have worked out our BMI (whether we are a healthy weight, overweight or obese) and our BMR (how many calories we should be consuming) and the physical activity levels we feel comfortable achieving, so what is next? Planning! I don't want you cutting down so drastically on your calories that you become nutritionally deficient, are unable to function or even worse, feel hungry all the time as then your lifestyle change will go out of the window. I want you to look at what your calorie intake should be and keep to it!

Here's a quick reminder:

Your body burns fuel (food) as calories
Any excess calories which are not burned are stored as fat
Fat is stored energy
Eating fewer calories than you need equals losing fat
Eating more calories than you need equals gaining fat

If your body burns 2,000 calories a day and you consume 1,500 calories a day, that is 500 calories per day or 3,500 calories per week, which will result in one pound of weight-loss.

Keep it simple! You will not fail if you follow the steps I have shown you regarding your BMI, BMR and activity levels. Here is an example:

Emily is 40 years old, 5 feet 5 inches tall and weighs 14 stone. She works in an office and drives there five days a week. Twice a week she goes to the gym and does thirty minutes exercise. Emily does not eat a healthy diet, she finds it easier to buy ready meals due to her work schedule. She enjoys the gym but she goes with her friend so she sees it as a social habit rather than an exercise workout. Emily wants to lose weight for her friend's wedding in a few months time and has spotted a lovely dress she would like to wear. So how can Emily do this?

Let us work out Emily's BMI – according to calculations on her gender, age, height and weight Emily's BMI is 32.6, meaning she is obese. Her activity levels are low because she drives to work and only does an hour of exercise a week, during which, as she admits, she spends most of the time chatting to her friend.

After calculating her BMR and using the Harris Benedict Formula I mentioned in an earlier chapter, she can work out her recommended daily calorie intake. Her BMR is 1625.1 and since she does little exercise her level is 1.2 so:

$$1625.1 \times 1.2 = 1,950 \text{ calories per day}$$

If her intake is more than this, she needs work out how to reduce it and think about how she can improve her activity levels if she wants to fit into that dress.

Now you have seen the example and worked out your BMI and BMR, let us work out a guide for you.

▪ Preparation

1. I have completed a guide I think will help you stay on track over the next few weeks. Firstly, write down the number of weeks over which you plan to lose weight and make a list of your goals.
2. Then think about the food you would like to be eating.
3. This is where your meal plans come in: planning your meals so that you balance your nutrients, calorie intake as well as your protein, carbs and vegetables will stop you reaching for a bar of chocolate or a bag of crisps.
4. The most important factor is which foods contain which nutrients and making sure they cover the five food groups.
5. This is your weight-loss journey, I am here to help you change your thinking around food and to hopefully influence you to a healthier and happier lifestyle.

You need to create an exercise and food chart. If you fill it in weekly you'll see your progress and your achievements.

WEEK ONE

- Record your weight and all your measurements and note this in a little book.
- Take a before picture of your body and put it in the book.
- You are now going to plan your meals for the week and make your shopping list.
- Buy your food for the week so you are not tempted to pop into supermarkets and remember to choose tasty meals you will look forward to.

You are going to write a list of the physical activities that you enjoy doing on your chart. Start off doing light exercise and see how you feel. Be kind to

Graphical planning and monitoring of daily meals

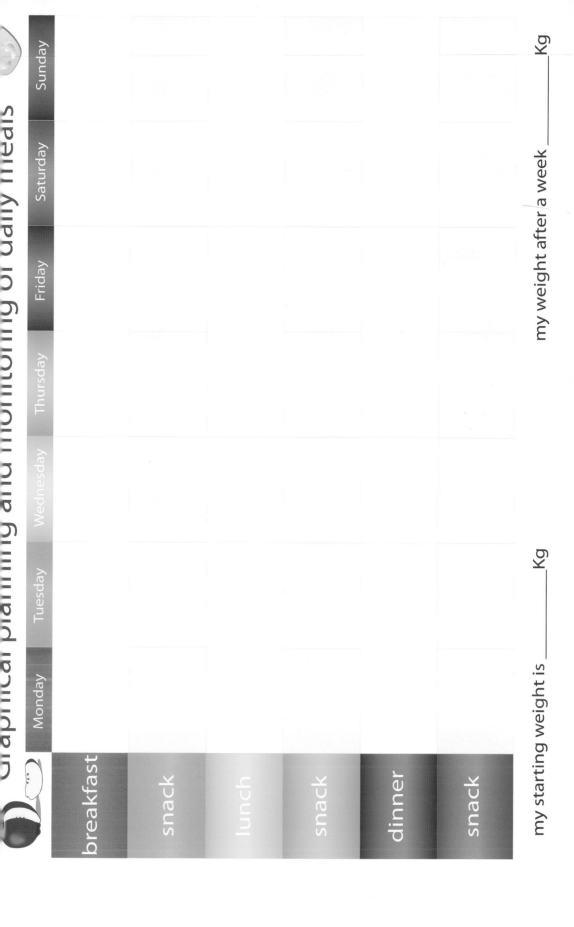

	Monday	Tuesday	Wednesday	Thursday	Friday	Saturday	Sunday
breakfast							
snack							
lunch							
snack							
dinner							
snack							

my starting weight is _____ Kg

my weight after a week _____ Kg

yourself: don't sign up for three hours of exercise a day if you aren't used to it: you'll give up. Try walking, going for a ten-minute jog or a swim. The government recommends that we spend a minimum of two and a half hours a week exercising so this is what you are aiming for if you are not there already.

WEEK TWO

- Plan your exercise. If you managed some exercise last week, try a bit more this week. Maybe go for something else. It's good to vary your routine as it stops you gets bored and it stretches other muscles. If you become sore or achy, take a bath or shower to soak them.
- Plan your meals and write your shopping list, sticking to healthy clean eating meals. Buy the food.
- Weigh yourself at the end of week and write this down.
- Fill in your activity chart.

WEEK THREE

- Look at other ways of exercising. If your work or children's school is within a good walking distance, ditch the car three times this week and walk to work. If you use public transport, then get off a stop earlier and walk the rest of the way to your destination.
- Research new healthy meals you can cook and enjoy.
- Ask friends would they like to join a gym or go for a run with you. If not, research activities you could do in a group where you will meet like-minded people – try yoga, Pilates, aerobics, Zumba, keep fit, aquarobics or maybe join a running or tennis club if you are already a bit more active.
- Plan your meals and shopping list. Buy the food.
- Fill in your activity chart.

WEEK FOUR

- Increase your exercise levels. Try a new physical activity twice this week.
- Plan your meals and shopping list and buy the food.
- Fill in your activity chart.
- Take measurements of yourself to see if you have lost any weight and write them down.

WEEK FIVE

- Plan your food and drink for the week and buy it.
- Maybe think about changing your snacks.
- Hopefully you are completing two sessions of exercise a week and have swapped your car for walking.
- Fill in your activity chart.

WEEK SIX

- Introduce another form of exercise which takes you to three sessions a week. These could be thirty minutes or hour sessions.
- Plan your meals and shopping list and buy the food.
- Write down your achievements so far and any goals you have met.
- Fill in your activity chart.

WEEK SEVEN

- Tell everyone about your new healthy lifestyle and how amazing you are feeling.
- Stick to your daily calorie intake but reward yourself with a treat.
- Plan your meals and shopping list and buy in the food.
- Continue to exercise.
- Fill in your activity chart.

WEEK EIGHT

- Plan a meal out with family or friends, this will test your willpower.
- Ensure you are completing at least two hours of exercise a week.
- Plan your meals and shopping lists.
- Look for some new healthy dinners you can create.
- Fill in your activity chart.
- Weigh yourself and take measurements.

WEEK NINE

- Write down everything you have enjoyed up until now.
- Write down what you have not enjoyed and think about how you could overcome this.
- Plan your meals and do your shopping from the list.
- Ensure you are completing the exercise sessions.
- Fill in your activity chart.
- Plan a treat for next week.

WEEK 10

- Well done – you have finished the first part of your healthy lifestyle journey and hopefully lost weight as well as increasing your exercise levels.
- Continue to fill in your activity chart until you feel comfortable you can do without it.
- Continue to plan your meals and shop weekly to avoid supermarket temptations.
- Continue with your exercise regimes.
- Visit your list about what you have enjoyed.
- Look at your weight and measurements along the way and look at how far you come and achieved.
- Weigh yourself.
- If you have not lost much weight re-evaluate your plan to what you could change. Did you really do the exercise you needed to do? Have you stuck to nutritious meals? Take an after photo of your body and compare to the before photo.

It is that easy. It is simply about changing your habits and mind set.

Positive thinking + eating better + exercise = FEELING GOOD and RESULTS Compare your food and drink intake before your diet to Week One of your diary log. Seeing the difference will help you feel more motivated. Below that is an example of a healthy eating plan. Remember that it is not just about cutting down on calories, it is about maintaining the right calorie intake for you and swapping high-fat, high-sugar, processed foods for low calorie natural ingredients. Bear in mind that if you are doing exercise, you may need more calories not fewer or you will be hungry.

Time	Type of food	Quantity	Calories (if known)	Additional information
8:30am	Cereal	1 3/4oz (50g)	140kcal	High sugar
	Milk – semi skimmed	3 1/2floz (100ml) approx	50kcal	
11.00am	Small apple		55kcal	
	Tea – tea sugar		1kcal	
	milk	1 cubedash	9kcal	
			10kcal	
12.30pm	Tuna sandwich			Low sat fat
	- bread	2 slices	184kcal	
	- tuna		43kcal	
	- mayonnaise		45kcal	
1.00pm	Packet of crisps	2.5oz (70g) bag	252kcal	High fat, high salt
6:10pm	Pasta salad	14oz (400g)	483kcal	
6.30pm	Cheese cake	1 slice	321kcal	High sugar
8.00pm	Crisps	2 bags	198kcal	High fat, high salt
10.00pm	Hot chocolate	1 large mug	199kcal	High sugar
	Total:		1933kcal	

Weekly example

Meal	Monday	Tuesday	Wednesday	Thursday	Friday	Saturday	Sunday
Breakfast	Muesli with skimmed milk	Fruit smoothie	Fruit and fibre with milk and strawberries	Kale and spinach smoothie	Porridge with fruit	Poached egg on wholegrain toast	Pancakes with fruit
Snack	Celery sticks	Orange	Rice cakes with hummus	Blueberries and raspberries	Unsalted nuts	Oatcakes	Yogurt
Lunch	Salad with boiled eggs	Sweet potato soup	Tuna pasta	Wholegrain pitta with chicken and salad	Salmon salad	Avocado and feta salad	Omelette with filling of choice
Snack	Banana	Cherry tomatoes and goats cheese	Apple	Vegetable sticks and hummus	Strawberries on wholegrain bagel	Tropical fruit parfait	Fruit kebabs
Dinner	Grilled chicken with baked sweet potato and veg	Poached salmon with asparagus, broccoli and kale	Vegetable stir fry	Green Thai curry with brown rice	Mushroom and spinach frittata with side dish	Turkey mince bolognaise with soft noodles	Pork chops and vegetables and potato of choice
Snack	Rice cakes and peanut butter	Boiled eggs	Unsalted nuts	Frozen yogurt with fruit	Unsalted popcorn	Kale chips	Seed mix

This is just one example of how you can vary your meals. Your recommended calorie intake will influence your meal and snack choices but I wanted to show you how your meal planning should look. Remember if you are having a meal the night before you could make extra and have the rest for lunch the next day. If you have leftover fruit why not make it into a delicious smoothie. Unused vegetables can be eaten as a snack with hummus or low fat cheese.

Weekends can be the hardest time to stick to your diet so build in a sweet snack or a treat so you don't feel like you're missing out. Just ensure it is within your calorie intake for that day.

EXCUSES AND HOW TO OVERCOME THEM

'I have eaten chocolate cake my diet is ruined.' No its not. This is called a minor setback. It will not ruin all the hard work you have done nor break the calorie bank. Put it behind you, stay positive and get back to healthy eating the next day. 'Help me, I cannot carry on.' If you feel like this then rewind to the way you felt when you started. Remember the reasons for beginning your weight-loss journey. Take a breather and have a night off. Negative thoughts will creep into you head, the key is how you approach and deal with them. Re-read the goals you set, if they are too challenging set mini ones that are achievable for you. If you feel stressed then the goals you set yourself are too high, bear in mind that your weekly goals do not have to focusing on weight-loss, they could be about introducing yourself to another form of exercise or cooking a new dish for you or the family. Stay positive and you will overcome the barriers. 'I cannot attend the gym tonight; my uncle's goldfish has passed away.' Making excuses is easily done but making weak excuses when you have worked so hard is foolish. The only way to adapt new habits and stick to them is by keeping your routine. If you choose to do fifteen minutes exercise instead of thirty, you will still have done some and some is better than none. 'I am exhausted; all this exercise is making me tired.' It is not called a workout for nothing. Exercise generates energy so gives you more of a boost than you need. If you feel that bad after exercise, take a look at the amount of time you are doing or the exercise itself, perhaps change it to something lighter and more manageable until you are used to the increased activity. You recharge your body through food, sleep and exercise. Movement creates energy. It gets your heart pumping, blood pumping, cleans out nasty toxins, and gets your engine started. It also gets confidence levels up so you feel better about yourself. Include all of this in your vision. You can do this! 'I am starving.' More often than not we actually mistake hunger for thirst. Try having a drink of water or a cup of tea before grabbing the chocolates. If you are still hungry, load up on snacks full of fibre; they're nutritious and filling, too. 'I don't have time to cook.' If you do not have time to cook, how do you suppose to eat? You cannot survive without eating so people make this excuse because they don't want to cook. It's not about time, if you have time to wait forty-five minutes for a takeaway to be delivered or thirty minutes for a frozen meal to finish cooking, you have time to cook a healthy meal and to be sitting there enjoying it. Make the time, prepare and plan. 'My cravings are out of control! I've eaten a packet of biscuits.' Your cravings are part of your habits. Humans are creatures of habit but we can change them. Our habits are our comfort zone and we do not like moving out of it. If you want to move out of your comfort zone you need to look at ways to improve your habits. You can use this as part of your preparation and goal setting. 'I have lost no weight this week – help.' Just because you have not lost weight does not mean the diet is not working, it means that your body is adjusting to your new way of life. Weight-loss is not a sprint, it is a marathon. You may not lose weight or inches one week but the week after you may lose double. It is about maintaining your journey, as I keep saying: do not weigh yourself weekly. We don't want any negative thinking which may give you a reason to quit. Stay positive and motivated. When you reach your ideal weight you are still going to need to maintain it so this excuse is just testing you for the rest of your journey.

Be consistent with your strongest healthy habits and be prepared to overcome your weaknesses.

Cooking methods

The way we cook our food also reduces the fat in our diets. For example, frying, particularly deep fat frying, uses lots of oil. If you are cooking fish or meat then try brushing the portions with oil rather than pouring the oil into the pan, this means you are using less oil. Try to use different cooking methods which are healthier. Here are some suggestions.

Braising – Involves cooking meat and veggies and usually herbs in little stock or water. Slow cookers are great for this if you want to cook a hearty soup or a home-made stew.

Poaching – No fat required with this cooking method as you poach eggs, fish, fruit or poultry in water or stock.

Stir-frying – Only a small amount of oil is needed so try using a healthy oil such as coconut. Stir-fry on a high heat and toss the food continuously to stop it from sticking and burning.

Grilling – This allows fat to drain away so it's great for cooking meats and fish. Line the grill pan with tin foil to cut down on cleaning and brush food with a little oil to prevent sticking. Grilling optimises the nutrients within food.

Steaming – Great for vegetables, fish and poultry and my main cooking method as it helps preserve the nutrients and it is quick and easy too.

Roasting – We all love a Sunday dinner with roast potatoes and meat. To ensure the fat is drained away put the food on a rack over a tray.

Microwaving – A quick way to cook veggies, not ready meals. Microwaving preserves nutrients and is great for reheating food you have pre-cooked and frozen.

Remember it is imperative that food is cooked at the correct temperature and for the right amount of time. Undercooking food can cause food poisoning if not cooked thoroughly.

Portion control

A serving and a portion are different things. Servings are recommended amounts of food and portions are the amount of food you choose to eat. Portion sizes are completely in your control – you can choose whether your portions are smaller or bigger than the recommended serving. For example, the label on a pack of cheese may advise that the cheese contains six servings, but the portion you choose to eat could be less than the recommended serving. You need to work out how you are going to use portion control within your diet so that you don't overload your plate.

Is organic better?

Organic foods are those grown without the aid of artificial chemicals and fertilisers, growth regulators and feed additives. With non-organic foods, the chemicals and pesticides can remain on foods after they have been harvested. Washing fruit and veggies, will remove some of these residues but not all and it can also remove some of the vitamins within the skins. This should not stop us eating them, some people choose to buy organic because they believe they are getting the complete goodness without the risk of consuming any of the chemicals. I prefer organic foods for a number of reasons though they are not for everyone, not least because they are more expensive:

- **Organic farmers are only allowed to use four pesticides out of the hundreds available.**
- **Independent research has shown consistently how organic food is higher in nutrients than traditional foods. Research shows that organic produce is higher in vitamin C, antioxidants, and the minerals calcium, iron, chromium, and magnesium.**
- **Organic foods are not allowed to contain hydrogenated fat.**
- **Any other additives are minimised.**

- They're free of neurotoxins that are apparently damaging to brain and nerve cells. Pesticides called organophosphates were initially developed as a toxic nerve agent during the First World War. When there was no longer a need for them in warfare, industry adapted them to kill pests on foods. Many pesticides are still considered neurotoxins.

- Genetically modified ingredients are not acceptable.

- Unless animals are ill, famers cannot use veterinary medicines on them so this decreases the chances of unwanted chemicals ending up in our bodies.

- Organic food is earth-supportive unlike modern farming practices, which can damage the environment through their use of pestcides and chemicals and their mass-production approach to farming.

- Studies have shown that organic foods may be higher in nutrients, however there are no long-term results.

- Organic food is often grown on small organic farms which helps support independent farmers.

People say that organic foods are more flavourful

Organic foods are not gas-ripened as some non-organic foods are (for example, bananas).

Organic farmers have high standards and are regularly inspected to meet organic compliance standards.

If you'd like to eat organic, you could have a go at growing your own fruit and vegetables; they would be more nutritious, more delicious and all that digging would keep you fit. Whether they're organic or not eating more fruits and vegetables is better for all of us. Do not let the organic/non-organic debate deter you: healthy nutrition is better than consuming processed foods full of salt and sugar.

We are nearly at the end of our book but this last chapter is here to show you what you need to do to stay positive and to ensure you maintain your weight-loss results. Remember that we all have slip ups and we all need a treat – it is how you manage these that counts. I hope this guide has helped you to put your own weight-loss plan together. What you need to remember is that this may be a slow process so do not make it slower by quitting.

CHAPTER 10

KEEPING MOTIVATED AND MAINTAIN RESULTS

'Believe you can and you are halfway there.'

Theodore Roosevelt

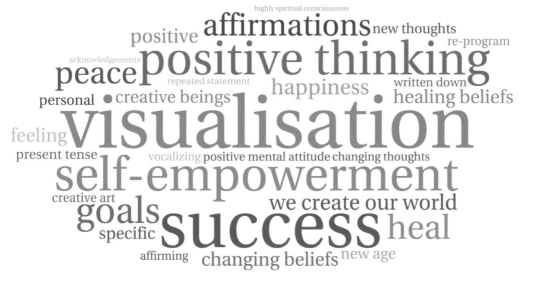

Positive quotes are my way of staying motivated no matter what goal I am trying to achieve. Positivity plays a significant role in our weight-loss efforts as it increases our motivation and our energy levels. Negative thoughts are self-defeating and lead to unhelpful behaviours such as skipping the gym, abandoning your diet and overeating.

Positive thoughts are encouraging. A negative attitude can set emotional processes and thoughts in train and that makes losing weight difficult. Berating yourself every time you eat the wrong foods, constantly focusing on what you cannot eat and approaching your exercise regime with dread are all ways that negative thought patterns can ruin your weight-loss efforts. When you hold a negative image of yourself, you deprive yourself of much-needed energy. When feeling incapable, depressed or unmotivated, it's easy to skip the gym or comfort eat to feel better. However, tuning into and acknowledging your feelings and transforming them into something more positive can actually help you achieve your weight-loss goals quicker. This is why I have suggested that you keep a diary. Once you write these feelings down and you acknowledge them, they have less power over you because your next step is to write a goal how to overcome them and then to write down how this negative feeling is actually a positive aspect about yourself.

As well as 'eat yourself thin', I want you to 'think yourself thin'. So here is what I want you to do: firstly I want you to write a list of the benefits of weight-loss - for example better health. Next work, write down a list of your best qualities. Now make a list of activities or things you like doing but don't have the time, this does not include eating! It could be listening to music, being pampered on a spa day, even cleaning. It is your list, so you pick. Write down a list of the naughty foods you enjoy and incorporate these into your healthy eating plan as a treat. Then think of ways you can make exercise fun. Picture doing the hoovering to music and dancing around the house. You are still burning calories. Or think how you could make the gym more fun such as by asking a friend to go with you. Next think of the positive ways you can get back on track after a slip up. If you slip up one day, don't dwell on it the next, just have a talk with yourself and counter your negative thoughts with positive ones. Finally, I want you to visualise what you would like to look like in a few months' time and how you want your lifestyle to be. This brings me to the next topic, the law of attraction.

THE LAW OF ATTRACTION AND WEIGHT-LOSS

You may be thinking: what on earth is the law of attraction? Let me explain: the law of attraction is the idea that by focusing on positive or negative thoughts a person will bring positive or negative experiences into their life. You may think this has nothing to do with weight-loss but it actually can overcome your negative thought processes about yourself. Let us experiment.

What do you see when you look in the mirror? Do you feel like you want to change something about yourself? Are you happy or upset or sad with what you see? Are you content with your lifestyle? Are you pleased with your activity levels? Your answers will probably be negative or you would not be reading this book. However, your answers can show how you could apply the law of attraction for weight-loss. Instead of focusing on problems such as your current weight and overeating as the problem, try focusing on the solution. Dissatisfaction with your weight is a negative thought. This single thought lies inactive in the brain until other negative thoughts spring up around it and you become swamped by a negative nightmare. But if negative thinking took just one thought to begin, it can be changed with just one positive thought. And this is what you are going to do.

Visualisation is a powerful tool for weight-loss. It connects the power of your mind, body and soul. Before you lose weight or accomplish any major goal, you must be able to see yourself doing it in your mind's eye. You use creative visualisation every day though you are probably unaware you are even doing it. When you daydream or create visions about food, people, clothes or anything else you want or aspire to, you are using creative visualisation.

Visualisation can focus your mind, improve your emotions, and provide powerful motivation and inspiration to keep you on track towards your weight-loss goals. Visualisation can help you manage stressful situations and keep you motivated when you are experiencing temptation, impulses and cravings.

Redirect your negative thoughts and focus on the aspects you like about yourself and the benefits of changing your lifestyle. Do not feel frustrated but appreciate that you are in good health and you are making this change for yourself to feel better. Replace your negative thoughts with positive ones by changing your perspective and addressing your inner patterns of thoughts and beliefs. If you love your body and you communicate that to the universe through positive images and visualisation, then the universe will reflect the truth back to you. So rather than focusing on what you are giving up, focus on what you will gain by losing weight. Do you think when a child learns to walk and falls down a hundred times, he thinks to himself 'maybe this isn't for me?' No he soldiers on, determined that he will walk. Think like this.

By visualising yourself as a slimmer and healthier individual, your subconscious mind will begin to believe you are this new person. Your subconscious mind will begin to aid and support you in achieving your goal. You will then begin to act in accordance with this new vision of yourself.

As you focus on your positive intention of losing weight through healthy eating and exercise, you will begin to attract experiences that are associated with your intention. You will feel more motivated to lose weight and to exercise or attend the gym. Experiences and people will show up around you to assist you in reaching your goal. You will find yourself more interested in healthy foods and you will feel the desire to exercise too.

Follow the steps I asked you to complete earlier and visualise each day how you want to look and this will help you on your weight-loss journey. A positive attitude will always receive positive results. The question is not who is going to let you fail, the question should be who is going help me achieve it? And the answer is YOU! Always start and end your day with a positive thought.

YOGA, MEDITATION AND RELAXATION

Relaxation

Relaxation is necessary for your mental and physical well-being. If you do not give yourself time to relax on a regular basis, your body and mind can become worn out and overwhelmed. Relaxation is the most natural and effective way to soothe and revitalize your mind. Through relaxation, you will become more in touch with your body, enabling you to recognize and overcome any tension more easily.

It's a discipline aiming to unite body, spirit and mind, helping oneself become more aware of their deepest natures!

Integrating a healthy nutritious diet and keeping active not only makes us look better on the outside, but makes us feel amazing from the inside. I want to do by doing it the RIGHT way!! Determination and discipline, knowing the difference between hunger and appetite, being aware of what you're eating and being active all play a huge role in creating a healthy lifestyle. I had a goal and was determined; I did cardio, weights and yoga to get my results. I pushed myself further every session and made myself get out of bed that extra hour early before work to do so.

Getting active first thing in the morning wakes you up immediately, sets you up for the day. It makes you feel great, boosts your metabolism, starts burning carbs and fat for fuel. By making a difficult decision so early in the day we are also strengthening our discipline and willpower, as well as our beautiful bodies. Of course, it isn't easy but what's more important than looking after our own body. It's the MOST important thing we own. Being fit is not just about looking good! It is about building our foundations and setting us up to live a longer and healthier life. We need muscle to protect our bones, as we get older our body starts to deteriorate. So making it stronger now will make life a lot less painful in the future. We don't have to be sweating it out in the gym or pumping through a class every spare hour we have, we just need to make small commitments and go for it. Once we achieve our results we can go further or slow down. But that's only if we do it the RIGHT way. I enjoy this lifestyle simply because I enjoy being active. The more we move, the more it becomes part of our lives and the more we will actually start to enjoy the benefits physically, mentally and emotionally. All these quick-fix diets, challenges and slimming pills are only temporary. Being fit and healthy is a long-term commitment not just a month of starving yourself to look good in a dress for one night. We all need to start somewhere and there's no point putting it off. Start looking after yourself today and feel the difference from within. No diet needs to start on Monday it can start any day of the week.

Yoga

'Yoga is an ancient science concerned with developing a holistic, healthy and harmonious way of living. It offers benefits that make the body stronger and healthier and calm the mind and soul. The word yoga has many shades of meaning, but is usually translated as the word 'union' and the practice can lead to the balance of our body, breath, mind and spirit.'

Yoga Scotland

My good friend, who is a yoga teacher, says; 'It's a discipline aiming to unite body, spirit and mind helping oneself become more aware of their deepest natures.'

Yoga has many benefits and it has become more and more popular around the world. If you do your own yoga practice then this is fantastic as I believe it helps so many people for so many reasons. The number of men doing yoga is increasing too and I genuinely believe it is a good way to replace any negative energy with positive thinking.

As I am not a yoga teacher I cannot talk about all the different types but what I can do is talk about yoga and weight-loss. As I have mentioned before stress causes us to eat a poor diet. Consumer Reports last year asked 1,328 psychologists which approaches are essential to losing weight and keeping it off, and the top answers were 'understanding and managing the behaviours and emotions' and 'emotional eating'. So it seems logical that a regular yoga practice, by improving how the brain controls your reaction to stress, could lead to healthier food choices and, perhaps, easier weight-loss. Not only will your mind benefit from practising yoga, it has been proven to help lose weight too. Research has shown in a study funded by the National Institutes of Health in the USA, women who did restorative yoga burned 2 per cent more body fat than those who just stretched for that same period of time. In another study in the Journal of Alternative Medicine, overweight men who practiced yoga and breathing exercises daily lost an average of four pounds in only ten days. Now this does not mean that each individual will lose this much but what it does prove is that yoga can help with weight-loss and positive thinking. This then brings me to meditation.

Would it be OK if every day you woke up feeling positive and happy about life? Would it be OK if you felt more relaxed? Would it be OK if you felt energised on a daily basis? Meditation can help you achieve these things. Weight-loss is not just about a change in eating habits it's about getting our minds to embrace healthy lifestyle changes and there is no better way than meditating. This centuries old practice has a positive impact on people and those who use it often report a happier life and an ability to tackle negativity head on. I know this from many of my friends who practice it. Sustainable weight-loss is not about tricking or forcing your body to be thin. It's about changing your body from the inside out so your body actually wants to be thin; you can do this by attending meditation classes within your area or looking at reliable sources online which can help you. The idea is to build healthy habits for life; you may quickly start to feel these positive affirmations and guided imagery being incorporated into your day-to-day consciousness. If you struggle with anxiety or are struggling on your weight-loss journey, or if you struggle with self-image, then meditation can help you along the way.

Mindfulness and Meditation

Mindfulness is a way of changing your relationships with the natural world, purposely focusing attention on the present moment, in a non-judgmental way. It will allow you to see things with more clarity, be calmer and understand yourself and others more compassionately. Mindfulness is a way of patiently having more moment-to-moment experiences, those we sometimes miss because we are too busy. It is a way of being more in touch with ourselves. It is not a passive way of interacting with our world, it provides clarity and wisdom and allows us to adapt, to be more flexible, and bring some creativity and spontaneity into our lives. It is an awareness of what is happening now, in the moment, and not being weighed down by the regrets of the past and worry of the future. Meditation is one of the best tools we can use to begin our mindfulness journey. Find a quiet and calm place, with no distractions, and begin to focus on your breathing. As you begin to breath, you will find that a whole lot of thoughts and feelings begin to arise. Once you have become aware of these thoughts and feelings, the process of awareness has begun. This is where mindfulness happens. As you become more aware of these thoughts and feelings, you should observe and not judge them. Accept them for what they are, which are just thoughts and ideas of the mind, and let them go. It is important to understand that mindfulness is not the answer to all your problems, but it will allow you to experience them in a whole new state: present moment of perspective with wisdom of insight. Strengthening your mindfulness is all about practice, the more you do the stronger you will become.

Stress within our minds

Most of the thinking we do involves pre-living events of the future or reliving past events. Playing visions and thoughts over in our minds making up stories to fit our perceptions of how things should have or might happen. We are attached to past situations that have no physical reality. These stick in the mind creating emotional and mental imbalances. Wanting, seeking and desiring are nothing but thoughts projected away from the now. A fundamental disagreement with the present moment: to want; is to say you are unhappy with what you already have, and seeking happiness in external things will only lead to more unhappiness within that moment. It's an embedded cycle of always wanting more, when really you don't 'need' anything to make you happy. If you always 'need' and always 'want', then you will never be satisfied. How many times do you say 'when I have this' or 'when I have achieved that', you will be happier and more joyful within your life. Then you receive it, and it is still not enough to keep a lasting sense of happiness. The truth is, that wanting happiness from the future doesn't exist, because we are always in the present moment, even though tomorrow is today's future, tomorrow will be tomorrow's present. Again, and again, and again. In the search for something to fill that sense of incompleteness we are living a story, our own story, and we will experience a whole lot of sensations along the way. But these sensations will come and go. They don't belong to us; they are strangers passing through the body at that moment in time. It's not for us to get rid of these feelings or hold on to them, but to learn to understand them and accept that the things that happen in life are not a part of who we are, they are just a part of the journey we choose to take. Everything in our lives right now is impermanent. Once we understand the true meaning of impermanence, only then we will truly accept the present moment. If you're thinking that this isn't for you, then this is fine too. We are all different and we do what works for us but being truly happy and positive within our selves will help us establish how we perceive our lives, others, our habits and how we view our new lifestyle change. Change does not come easy. Remember you have always been beautiful, but now you are just deciding to become healthier, fitter, faster and stronger! Remember that always!

So I have spoken about ways to think positive so here are some of my top tips to losing weight; note this down as this can help you along the way. These top tips are everything we have discussed throughout the book, but repeating them in a short and simple format may improve your way of remembering them.

TOP TIPS FOR LOSING WEIGHT

Meals

Keep meals simple. If you enjoy cooking and you are loving all the new recipes and creating new meals then this is great, continue with this, but if you're finding it time-consuming then keep food simple. Healthy eating does not need to be complicated.

Eating habits

Eat meals and snacks regularly to beat cravings and fill up on fruits and vegetables, which will make you feel fuller. Continue to eat breakfast, it will help you maintain a better weight-loss in the long run. Make salads chunky so you feel fuller and do the same with cooked veggies.

Cravings

If you get a craving for foods, then have something sweet to take away the taste or try chewing gum. Do not ignore your cravings or you may give in to a different type of sweet snack which will leave you feeling deflated.

Planning

Planning your meals and shopping lists will save you time over the rest of the week. Especially if you are preparing your meals and freezing them. So if you are short of time on one day you will have a healthy meal in the freezer ready to pop in the oven. If you have children ask them to help you prepare packed lunches, this involves them and encourages them to support you on your lifestyle change. They may even benefit too.

Stocks

Always ensure your cupboards are well stocked. This could mean getting rid of any junk food and replacing it with dry and tinned foods that you could use to whip up a quick and tasty nutritious meal. What I mean by dry foods are brown rice, pasta and a variety of herbs. Tinned foods include tuna, salmon and mackerel, tinned low-salt baked beans, beans and pulses. Keep your freezer full too with meals you have frozen and frozen food you have bought such as fish, veggies and fruits which are also a great way to eat healthy if you are in a hurry.

A freezer also costs less to run when full rather than when it's half empty.

Shop smart

Use the traffic light system and all the labelling advice I have given you. Once you have mastered the art of food labelling you will just become used to purchasing the new health foods as part of your weekly shop. Look for offers and vouchers and shop around to find the best deals. If you have access to independent shops or farmers' markets go there as you're buying fresher produce while supporting local businesses and farmers.

Don't get confused

Four ways you can avoid being misled through selective information and labelling

Natural – People hear the word natural and automatically assume this means healthy, when in fact the products may be natural but also may have a very high-fat or sugar content.Information on calcium, iron and vitamins. Two concerns here: firstly the food may contain vitamins or minerals but the quantities may be minute; secondly the food may contain these nutrients, but it may also contain higher levels of fat or sugar.

Reduced fat – The food may be lower in fat but it still does not necessarily mean that the rest of the product is healthy. And lower in fat is not the same as low-fat.

Wholegrain – The wholegrains in cereals may be high in, say, cereal but the levels of sugar may also be higher and the amount of processed wheat and flour may be greater.

Always check the contents to avoid being misinformed.

Let's look at some tips for exercising and let's be excited to start. Being fit isn't a fad or a trend it is a healthy lifestyle.

TOPS TIPS FOR EXERCISING

Choose an activity you will enjoy

If you hate running, then you would not pick running as your first choice of exercise. As there are so many types of exercise, you don't have to do one you don't enjoy. This isn't an inconvenience or a duty, it's a hobby and one which will keep you fit and healthy. If you're struggling to think of ideas, then look at local community groups, which may offer a range of activities, or local gyms that offer new classes. Many local authority gyms have programmes specially designed for people who are new to exercising.

If you enjoy what you do, then that's half the battle. If you hate your job then it becomes a chore, you don't enjoy going, you lack motivation. Exercise is the same. Keep it fun.

Plan it

If you keep focused and add exercise into your plan, then you have no excuse not to go. It's too easy to think you will go after work and then find an excuse not to. Why not try sticking to the same time each week so you have a routine you can look forward to. You could even do exercises before work, which will give you an additional energy boost for the day, and also put you in a better mood. Try to avoid exercise just before bed as this may leave you feeling energised and stop you sleeping. Not a good idea.

If you build this into your plan, then you will start to visualise it and a structure will form within your day. This makes it easier to create a healthy lifestyle and also gives you the enthusiasm to stick at it. *Vary your exercises.*

As well as choosing an activity you will enjoy, find a broad range of activities to do. Try new adventures: maybe a walk in another city, hiking up Snowdonia, gymnastics and kick boxing, maybe even salsa lessons. Either way keep it varied. I love running and running outdoors but I choose to do this on my own rather than in a group. I also enjoy doing home workouts such as Zumba and aerobic exercises as this suits me. You could be the opposite and choose to have people around you for motivation. I enjoy yoga with friends as I find this helps me banish any negative energy. All these things fit in around my schedule and work commitments so it's a win-win situation for me. It is about doing what suits you, what you are comfortable with and knowing your boundaries. Keeping exercise varied keeps the fun and excitement in and makes you determined to keep up a healthy way of life.

It can be cheap

Don't think that you need to go out and purchase the top of the range equipment or join an expensive gym or hire a personal trainer. Exercise can be free. Many gyms now also offer no sign-up fees and you can attend their classes paying when you go. Make use of the lovely parks within your area or do it all from the comfort of your own home. Keep it basic to start with and you will soon think of new and exciting activities and cheap and cheerful ways do them.

Stick with it

Once you have reached your target weight continue with your exercise. Don't think because you have lost the weight that you will stay that weight. Constancy equals results and after coming so far to change your lifestyle why would you want to go back. Why not look and feel this good all the time. If you are having a down day then still carry on, exercise can often help you feel better. So if you don't feel like going to the gym, try a workout at home or a more calming exercise such as yoga or mediation. There are always alternatives and choices to make. You are in control.

What you need to remember is that this is not the end. This is the start of your new healthy lifestyle and it is down to you to continue on your journey.

Maintaining results is going through everything we have spoken about within this book. So let us remind ourselves what I have hopefully helped you achieve.

Stick to the low calories – Your efforts will be showing on your waistline and in your health, so stick to the low calorie food and drink and don't give in to temptation. Continue to eat breakfast and don't slip into old habits of skipping it. Keep reminding yourself that breakfast gives you nutrients not empty calories. Continue with your food and activity charts so you can visualise what you are consuming.

Weighing yourself – By all means weigh yourself but don't do it weekly. Maybe go for once every two weeks or once a month. Keeping up the exercise and healthy eating will help you continue on your journey. Do the measurements and focus on what fits you now such as shoes, boots, underwear, jeans and even your wedding ring.

Planning – Being organised is one of the best assets to have when losing weight. Plan everything from your shopping lists to your meals to your exercise regime. Plot holidays and special occasions on a calendar and think about what you will eat and how you will stay on track!

Achievements - Always remember to reward your achievements. This does not mean eat a cream bun or completely destroy your diet, it means buy yourself a new book or CD with the money you have saved by not eating takeaways or junk food. Visual results will keep you focused so use the before and after photographs you took and pin them somewhere you can see them so that when you are having a down day, you can look at these and feel proud. There is no better feeling than knowing you have achieved something. By now people will be complimenting you on how great you look which will keep you smiling, happy and strong-minded.

Support – Do not forget that you still need support. So keep like-minded people around you and their positivity will keep you going. You don't want negative nellies surrounding you. You may get snide comments from jealous people but remember jealousy is just a lack of self-confidence and keep smiling – it confuses them. Surround yourself with a circle of friends, family and gym buddies and don't forget the biggest tool, social media, which is full of groups on the same journey. It's a great way to connect with people and give each other the inspiration and determination you need and deserve. I have said it before, and will say it again: keep some positive quotes to inspire and keep you in a happy frame of mind, read motivational articles and book on the law of attraction. Remember every day is a new day, a fresh start and a new beginning, embrace this and ignore people who say it can't be done. They should not be interrupting those who are doing it.

Enjoy the change – Welcome your new healthy lifestyle and take pleasure from it. Whether you enjoy your new nutritious diet, the cooking or even the exercise, make sure your weight-loss journey is enjoyable or you are more likely to fail. And we don't do failures on this programme, we love triumphs and the compliments we get from people about how well we look.

Overcoming obstacles – This ties in with the planning but remember challenge is what makes life more interesting and overcoming them gives us the best satisfaction in the world. If plan A does not work, don't worry. Just remember the alphabet has twenty-five more letters.

New habits – Now you have kicked all your old habits out of the window, keep them there. You have learned new ways to control your emotions around food so stay consistent. Keep reminding yourself of your new habits and keep implementing new goals to aim for and achieve. If, at work, you regularly go for lunch a friend then suggest you both bring a packed lunch and eat it in the park, then breaking an old habit and introducing a new one. Plan your next move because every step contributes to your goal.

Think like a winner – Because that is what you are. Believe it and achieve it. You are in control all the time and you have succeeded just by trying. The first step was purchasing this book and that's a success in itself.

Limit your time – Limit your time on technology. Rather than spending the evening browsing social media, keep up your hard work doing some outside exercise or go to the gym. Technology has taken over our lives but sometimes it is nice to have a break from the latest status on social media or the soaps on TV. Think about ways to exercise while talking on your phone, putting the laundry out, cleaning and dusting, every little bit helps to tone you and to lose weight. If you cannot drag yourself away from your regular television show, do exercises in front of it. At least get up to switch channels instead of hitting the remote. Imagine how many times you would do that through the evening.

Put your phone to good use – I have spoken about spending less time on your phone but this might actually help those of you who have their phones glued to their hands. Smart phone applications have never been so popular; you can get an app for almost anything including visualisation techniques, positive affirmations and exercise apps and logs. There are others related to weight-loss and healthy lifestyles and I was shocked to learn you can even download one regarding your toilet habits. Here some types of apps I have come across:

- **Personal trainer apps which assess your fitness levels after each workout. They do this by asking you a serious of questions which determines your fitness levels and then reassessing after each workout.**

- **You can download apps for workouts, exercises, running and even muscle and body building which follow the same principles.**

- **This one was a big surprise to me: there's an app which uses the camera on** your phone and measures how well you keep up with the workout. I found this a little creepy to think a stranger could be watching me.

- Training for a marathon? Download the app which completes training plans for you.

- Can't measure your speed or distance? There's an app to help you track it.

- Food and activity log? Who needs good old-fashioned pen and paper when you have an app to hand to do this for you.

- Confused with calories? An app will count the calories in your food diary.

- Suffer with allergies? There's an app to tell you all about the foods you can and can't eat.

- Struggling to find healthy restaurants in your area? Download an app to help you.

- Mind and brain apps were new ones to me but ones I found interesting. Keeping track of your goals via an app is a good way to stay focused.

- There are apps for mediation and yoga so you can learn from your own home.

- You can even monitor your sleep patterns with an app.

- As always with anything on the internet, be careful when downloading these apps. Ensure they are from trusted and reliable sources and always check the ratings from previous users. A low rating means it is just wasting precious storage space on your phone but a high rating means it may of use to you. Pen and paper or new technology, it's up to you. Find the way which is easiest and gets you results. This is your weight-loss journey after all.

Bullet point tips

I have discussed the main tips above on what you can do to stay focused. Let us summarise the whole book in bullet points to ensure you succeed on your new path.

- Limit calorie intake

- Exercise frequently

- Plan and review your goals weekly

- Look at positive quotes

- Don't use excuses to skip the gym

- Plan smart – holidays and special occasions can't be used as excuses every week

- Don't weigh weekly

- Take measurements

- Drink plenty of fluids (in particular water)
- Fill up on veggies
- Create new meals
- Vary your diet
- Stop eating junk food
- Eat fresh not processed
- Eat breakfast
- Pack a lunch
- Ditch the old habits
- Stay active
- Monitor your progress
- Reward yourself with treats
- Cut up food – apparently can trick your brain into thinking you're eating more
- Know the difference between a portion and a serving size
- Watch out for alcohol – it's just liquid calories
- Use friends and family for motivation
- Don't be tempted by the latest quick fix fad diet
- No negative thoughts allowed
- Snack right
- Shop smart
- Love yourself
- Try new activities
- Spice up your meals
- Check out alternative therapies which may help with stress – for example, yoga and meditation
- Set new goals weekly
- Join local weight-loss communities
- Enjoy watching your progress in the mirror
- Visualise all you would like to achieve
- Keep on top of your food and exercise diary
- Spread the positivity by letting everyone know how well you're doing
- Stay motivated – You are a powerful and beautiful person and destined for great things

'EMBRACE THE JOURNEY'

Don't ever let anyone tell you that you can't, do not be deterred by negative thinking, do not think you have failed by a minor setback or slip up, stay motivated and consistent, achieve your goals and hit new targets, plan your adventure so you stay on track and always believe in yourself.

You can achieve what you believe and in a few months from now you will thank yourself.

Conclusion

I would like to thank you for reading my book and wish you the best of luck on this new adventure. I hope in some way I've inspired you to take a new approach to the way you think, whether it is thinking more positively, changing your lifestyle or giving you that push to try new activities, hobbies or even recipes, I will be happy to think it has helped in some way. When you feel like quitting, remember why you started. Re-read this book if you need to. I feel this book is different to other weight-loss books – I wanted to relate to you as an individual and to make you feel like we are on this journey together. The book was based on facts, studies, medical resources, professional guidance and personal experience and I wish you every success in the future on your journey and changes that you make. Remember when you lose that weight, or you are in the gym singing away to your favourite song, or maybe cooking a new healthy recipe in the kitchen, then look back and think of this book and say 'I ate myself thin'.

Keep me updated on your new adventures and remember: this is not the end, it is just the beginning.

Thank you and good luck x

REFERENCES

Achaya, K.T. *Indian Food: A Historical Companion* Delhi: Oxford University Press, 1994.

Appleby P.N., Thorogood M., Mann J.I., Key T.J.. (1999) *The Oxford Vegetarian Study: An Overview*. Am J Clin Nutr.70 (suppl): 525S–531S.

Bijlefeld, Marjolihljn. *Encyclopaedia Of Diet Fads*. Westport, CT, Greenwood Press, 2003. 242 p.

Booher, James Mathew, M.D., ed. *Scientific Weight Control; an improved system for reducing or increasing weight, together with an explanation of the benefits to be gained from weighing daily*. Chicago Continental Scale Works, 1925. 104 p.

Bundesen, Herman Niels. *Your Greatest Wealth Is Health*. Chicago, Shrewesbury Publishing Co., 1928

Clemens, R. and Pressman, P. and technologists (2005). Detox Diets Provide Empty Promises. *Food Technology*. (59/5). 18

Foxcroft, Louise. *Calories & Corsets: A History Of Dieting Over 2,000 Years*. Profile Books, London, 2011. 232

Gratzer, W.B. *Terrors Of The Table: The Curious History Of Nutrition*. Oxford University Press, Oxford 2003

Harvard's Women's Health Watch (2008). The Dubious Practices Of Detox: Internal Cleansing May Empty Your Wallet, But Is It Good For Your Health? Harvard Medical School, 2008

Hirst, Mike. *Germany*. Austin, TX: Raintree Steck-Vaughn, 2000. www.foodineverycountry.com
Hospodar, Miriam Kasin. *Heaven's Banquet: Vegetarian Cooking for Lifelong Health The Ayurveda Way* E.P. Dutton, New York, 1999.

Jaffrey, Madhur. *Madhur Jaffrey's Spice Kitchen*. Carol Southern Books, New York, 1993.

Passmore, Marian. *Fit For Kings: A Book Of Recipes*. Bruton, England: King's School, 1994.Black P.H. and Garbutt L.D. Stress, Inflammation And Cardiovascular Disease. Journal Of Psychosomatic research, 2002

Popkin, B.M., D'Anci, K.E. & Rosenberg, I. H. (2010) Water, Hydration And Health. *Nutrition Reviews*, 68(8), pp.439–458.

Ritz, P. & Berrut, G. (2005) The Importance Of Good Hydration For Day-to-day Health. *Nutrition Reviews*, 2005. 63(6 Pt 2): S6-13.

Sacks F.M., Bray G.A., Carey V.J., et al. *'Comparison Of Weight-loss Diets With Different Compositions Of Fat, Protein And Carbohydrates'*. N. Engl. J. Med. 2009 360 (9): 859–73.

Schwartz, Hillel. *Never Satisfied: A Cultural History Of Diets, Fantasies And Fat*. Free Press, New York. Collier Macmillan, London.

Classic British: Authentic And Delicious Regional Dishes. Smithmark, New York. 1996

https://www.gov.uk/government/statistics/national-diet-and-nutrition-survey-results-from-years-1-to-4-combined-of-the-rolling-programme-for-2008-and-2009-to-2011-and-2012

Related materials

Granberg, Ellen. 'Is That All There Is?' Possible Selves, Self-change And Weight-loss. *Social Psychology Quarterly*, v. 69, June 2006: 109-126.

Green, Andrew J. Fox, Kathleen, M., and Grandy, Susan. Impact Of Regular Exercise And Attempted Weight-loss On Quality Of Life Among Adults With And Without Type 2 Diabetes Mellitus. *Journal Of Obesity*, v. 2011 (3).

Hayenga, Elizabeth Sharon. *Dieting Through The Decades: A Comparative Study Of Weight Reduction In America As Depicted In PopularLiterature And Books From 1940 To The Late 1980s*. University of Minnesota, 1988. 678 p.

Jou, Chin. *Controlling Consumption: The Origins Of Modern American Ideas About Food, Eating And Fat, 1886-1930.*Princeton University, 2009. 261 p.

Jutel, Annemarie. Does Size Really Matter?: Weight And Values In Public Health. *Perspectives In Biology And Medicine*, v. 44, spring 2001: 283-296.

La Berge, Ann F. How The Ideology Of Low Fat Conquered America. *Journal Of The History Of Medicine And Allied Sciences*, v. 63, Apr. 2008: 139-177.

Martin, Corby K., O'Neil, Patrick M., and Binks, Martin. An Attempt To Identify Predictors Of Treatment Outcome In Two Comprehensive Weight-loss Programs. *Eating Behaviors*, v. 3, autumn 2002: 239–248.

Miller-Kovach, Karen. *She Loses, He Loses: The Truth About Men, Women And Weight-loss*. Hoboken, NJ, John Wiley & Sons, c2007. 242 p.

World Health Organisation (WHO) www.who.int

International Diabetes Federation (IDF) www.idf.org

The UN Food and Agriculture Organisation Food Balance Sheets faostat3.fao.org

The Organisation for Economic Cooperation and Development (OECD) www.oecd.org/united kingdom

External reading

British heart foundation www.bhf.org.uk

Harvard medical www.health.harvard.edu

Help guide to mental health and well being www.helpguide.org

NHS resources www.nhs.uk

Nutrition.gov www.nutrition.gov

The American Journal Of Nutrition ajcn.nutrition.org/

Resources

Counselling directory

www.counselling-directory.org.uk/

Nutritional therapy United Kingdom

bant.org.uk/bant/jsp/practitionerSearch.faces

Public Health England

www.gov.uk/government/organisations/public-health-england

The British wheel of yoga

www.bwy.org.uk/

The Institute For Complementary And Natural Medicine

icnm.org.uk

INDEX